A Father's Report

"My four Lamaze babies have convinced me that there is a great need for trained fathers. Donna and I began our Lamaze classes when she was seven months pregnant. Almost immediately I was able to help with Donna's breathing and especially her relaxation patterns.

"There was something rewardingly different about this way of having babies. I was aiding my wife and learning how to help her through labor and delivery. By the time our baby was due we were both elated about the prospects.

"The challenge of childbirth provides many men with an opportunity to establish mature, deep relationships with their wives. In this time of stress, a husband's active participation demonstrates that he cares a good deal about what is happening to the woman he loves. He assumes responsibility toward both his wife and the child they have conceived. Nothing can replace the intimacy and richness of sharing which a trained husband can impart at childbirth."

—Rodger Ewy

Preparation for Childbirth

A Lamaze Guide by
Donna and Rodger Ewy

THIRD EDITION

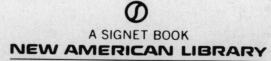

A SIGNET BOOK
NEW AMERICAN LIBRARY
TIMES MIRROR

PUBLISHER'S NOTE

The ideas, procedures, and suggestions contained in this book are not intended as a substitute for consulting with your physician. All matters regarding your health require medical supervision.

First Signet Printing, June, 1972
Ninth Signet Printing (Second Edition), December, 1976
Fourteenth Signet Printing (Third Edition), December, 1982

14 15 16 17 18 19 20 21 22
PRINTED IN THE UNITED STATES OF AMERICA

To Marguerite, Suzanne, Rodger, and Leon

Contents

8

Preparation for Childbirth

Foreword

As soon as I saw Donna and Rodger Ewy's manuscript, before even reading it, I agreed to write this Foreword. This quick decision may seem surprising, but let me explain. While the Ewys lived in France, I had the opportunity to meet them and talk with them, to exchange ideas, and to admire Rodger Ewy's photographic talents. I used one of his beautiful photographs in my book, *Childbirth with Confidence*.

Before reading this book, it was evident to me that they not only understood the method, but could also present it in human terms, in the spirit of its proponents. I was convinced that, because of their own personal experiences, they would be able to describe the unique experience of childbirth with intelligence, tact, and honesty. After reading this book, my impressions are confirmed.

Having learned about the method in France, the Ewys had the good fortune to meet several concerned doctors in Denver and to arouse the interest of Sister Margaret-Ann. By working with these people and by learning from their professional competence, the Ewys were able to avoid the basic errors which certainly would have given rise to criticism. Medicine is always critical of those who write concerning the art!

The great merit of this book is that it is directed to the general public, written in language which all will understand. It is the authors' real-life experience, analyzed and presented in simple terms.

I do not intend to give a complete analysis of this book. That would be unnecessary, and would rob the book of its savor. There are certain points of detail, in particular those which concern the different types of breathing, which may differ slightly from ours, and the emphasis on physical exercises is greater than we generally give. But it is the general principle and the goal that matter; each is free to use his personal approach.

In reading this book, I especially appreciated the analysis of the roles of the mother-to-be and her husband. We feel that the presence and participation of the husband, both during pregnancy and during labor and delivery, are of the greatest importance, for the emotional and practical assistance he provides.

In France there are specially trained "monitrices" who assist the woman during labor and delivery; because there are no such women in the United States, the husband's presence is indispensable. Thus, he should also be educated and informed, to be a director and a support for his wife.

It is fortunate that a couple can express their own reactions in such a unique situation. I find the tables which outline these roles (pp.161-68) particularly effective—so much so that I would not hesitate to use them as examples with my own patients.

In conclusion, I hope that this book will be read by pregnant women and their husbands, and also by doctors and medical personnel not yet familiar with the psychoprophylactic method of childbirth. They will find here the indispensable elements for successful childbirth, and will understand the reasoning of the authors, who share our fundamental concepts: to provide maximum safety for the mother and for the child, while respecting the intimate relationship of the parents and humanizing obstetrical technique.

To all those who have contributed to this book, I extend the grateful admiration of myself and my colleagues who, throughout the world, are striving to obtain the same goal. The psychoprophylactic method of obstetrics undeniably represents a victory of knowledge over ignorance, of activity over passivity, of man over animal. This is what those who have con-

tributed to publishing the book have understood and
conveyed.

Pierre Vellay, M.D.

Pierre Vellay, M.D.
Secretary of the International Society for
Psychoprophylaxis in Obstetrics
Paris, France

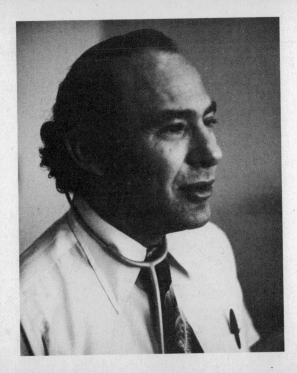

Foreword

Rodger and Donna Ewy are exciting people. They have enthusiasm, and the ability to convey their enthusiasm to others. In their classes they teach much more than preparation for childbirth—they also teach dignity and self-assurance.

Most obstetricians would agree that the ideal patient is one who is knowledgeable about labor, eager to give birth, and cooperative—and one who requires a minimal amount of analgesic and anesthesia. This is the ideal that the Ewys strive for.

For over fifteen years, I have encouraged my patients to take instructions in prepared childbirth. It is difficult to evaluate the results, but I think I can make some observations. Educated childbirth, as I prefer to call the method, gives the patient a good understanding of the birth process. She is familiar with most of the terms used, and therefore we can discuss more intelligently any problems that arise.

There is more cooperation on the part of the trained patient. Her husband is more involved and more knowledgeable. In a research study sponsored by the University of Colorado we are now attempting to measure, scientifically and exactly, the medical benefits of preparation, such as reduction in the need for drugs and reduction in the duration of labor. We anticipate positive results.

As a doctor, I oppose many "methods" of childbirth because of the rigid systems they present. The teachers of these methods often develop a fanatic attachment to the system for its own sake, rather than for the ultimate goal of a healthy mother and baby.

The Ewys are able to teach educated childbirth as a tool to help the patient through labor and delivery directed by the doctor. I, as an obstetrician, meet no resistance or sense of failure on the part of the patient when medication or surgical intervention is indicated.

Donna and Rodger Ewy have made a valuable contribution in our community, and this book should extend that contribution to a wider audience.

Harvey Cohen, M.D.
Diplomate of the American College of Obstetrics and Gynecology

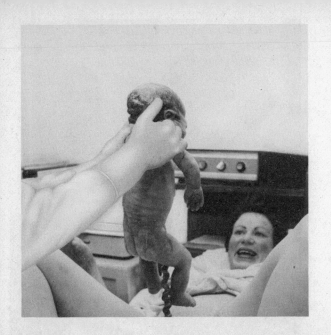

Preface

This is a book on childbirth, written by laymen for laymen in laymen's terms. It was not written for doctors or nurses; there are other fine books written by and for them. It is only for you, the bewildered mother- and father-to-be, from two who were also bewildered by the disconcerting technicality of what little material is available to the average person interested in childbirth.

We are becoming an increasingly educated populace. The parents of today are far more educated than any generation in history. Many husbands and wives are no longer content to be passive participants in the birth of their babies. They want to know not only what happens physically, but also how they are going to respond to the challenges of childbirth.

This book is dedicated to those of you who want to assume an active role in the birth of your child. Just as you can learn the proper way to read, drive, or ski, so you can learn the effective way to give birth.

In the following chapters you will learn not only what happens during birth but also techniques to use during labor and delivery that will help you work with, rather than against, the normal process of childbirth.

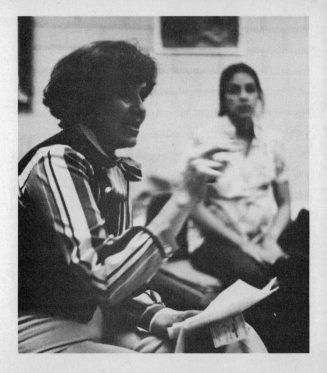

Chapter One: Introduction

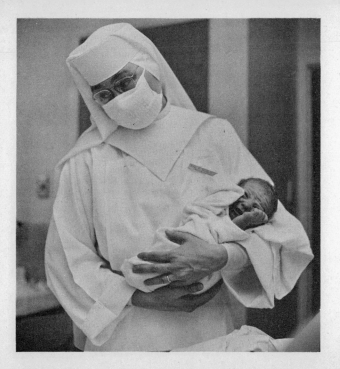

Sister Margaret-Ann, Supervisor of Obstetrics at St. Anthony's Hospital in Denver, assisted in the birth of our baby and described with beautiful simplicity the meaning of Lamaze:

> I shall always cherish the memory of the greatest moment of my obstetrical life. The creation of a new being was intended to be a soul-inspiring cooperation at the moment of birth, not only at the moment of conception. Would that more couples were able to appreciate this privilege and regard it as such.

This sensitive observation from a nurse who had participated in thousands of deliveries was inspired by the birth of our third child through the Lamaze method.

Like so many other important events in life, our introduction to Lamaze occurred much by chance. We had decided after our marriage to set a course for

Europe. Our parents thought we were mad to give up our jobs, sell all our earthly possessions, and take off for points unknown to work as photojournalists. But we knew that with Rodger's background in architecture and engineering and mine in education we would always be able to pursue those professions, and Europe offered so much to experience and enjoy.

We spent the first three years traveling throughout Europe, making photographs, and writing stories; studying castles, cathedrals, cuisines, and customs. Our business flourished, and the subject of childbirth could not have been further from our minds. But after three memorable years of travel and work, several mornings of nausea and a missed menstrual period made it evident that we had accomplished the feat of conceiving a child. We were delighted. It certainly was time we "settled down" and started our family.

However, I found that my ignorance about delivering children was appalling. I knew that my moth-

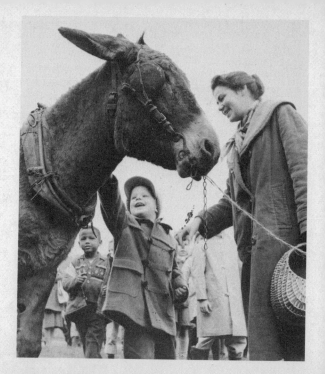

er's experiences had been horrendous. Through the years stories told by my friends had left a picture of pain associated with childbirth. From movies and novels images of agonizing moans, clenched fists, and painful cries lingered—quite a negative collection of impressions with which to start.

Although this painted a rather dreary picture, I still wasn't too concerned with the pain factor. However, the thought of losing my self-control and dignity during birth was distinctly distasteful, as I felt somehow that birth should be a positive, creative experience.

During the latter part of our stay in France, I had assumed the organization of a kindergarten at a nearby American Air Force Base. Being employed on an American base, I was eligible for Uncle Sam's maternity benefits. I looked forward to my first doctor's appointment, hoping that my fears and ignorance would be dispelled.

Although the waiting lines for maternity patients were long, I found chatting with my colleagues-in-waiting quite enlightening. The "experienced" prenatal patients found ready listeners among us novices, and the pains and aches of pregnancy and childbirth flowered in the teeming, steaming waiting room. When I finally did get in to see the doctor, I found that I hardly knew how to put my questions into words. As he was very busy, he had neither the time nor the patience to help me, and it was a very frustrating experience.

I went directly to the library, determined to be equipped with more knowledge so that I could express myself. As I pored over the books, it became evident how very little I knew about this important thing that was happening to me. It was incredible to me that through twenty-eight years of living, including four years of college and five years of teaching, I had learned so little about childbirth. On the next meeting with the doctor, I went armed with my list of "unknowns." As he examined me, he threw out a few technical answers in an impersonal way. With a final pat on the back he told me not to "busy my little head" with all those questions. "Don't you worry about a thing. We'll take care of you and give you a fine little baby." As I walked from his office, I found that the concept of his "giving" me my baby was rather disappointing, and it was then that I determined to find another answer.

Both Rodger and I began to delve more deeply into the subject of childbirth. One of the books we happened to pick up was Dr. Grantly Dick-Read's *Childbirth without Fear*. His positive, humane attitude was a very welcome one for us. How refreshing to read that childbirth need not be an unbearable experience but a simple, joyful, and natural act. We were grateful for Dick-Read's positive approach; however, there remained many unanswered questions, particularly about the actual birth. We re-read the book to see if we had missed some vital points on our first eager reading, but we could find nothing that explained what the woman would be doing during the birth to make such an experience possible. Dick-Read's method, bordering on mystical acceptance, seemed intellectually unsatisfying.

In the neighboring village of Chauny a close French friend of ours, Ghislaine Berlemont, lived; she worked as a physiotherapist. We broached the subject of childbirth to her. By an unusual coincidence, she was being employed by the French government to teach Lamaze childbirth classes in her village. "Would we be interested in visiting her classes?"

The next Wednesday Rodger and I walked into her class, curious to find out what this Lamaze method was. Ghislaine was explaining the principles of the method:

> The Lamaze technique not only recognizes the psychological aspects of childbirth, but also gives you techniques to use which will help you to work with your labor and delivery. By making a team of your educated mind and trained body, you will be able to

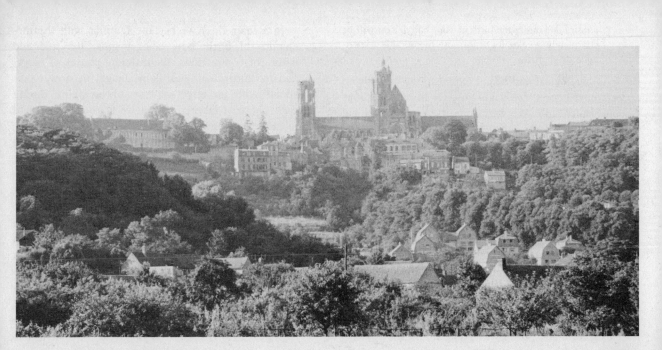

control and direct the birth of your baby. You will be completely awake for this most memorable experience of your life.

As her logical and sound explanations developed, we found honest, forthright answers to our questions concerning birth. We were impressed by the rational and scientific approach. Enrolling in her classes, we began our richly fulfilling association with the Lamaze method. The first class we attended acquainted us with its philosophy, history, and goals. The next lesson provided a thorough insight into women's physiological and mental processes. Together we learned how the baby develops from conception to birth and how my body was made to cope with the growth and actual birth.

Ghislaine then showed us how the muscles when tensed can cause discomfort during the birth and how, by relaxing these muscles, a woman can alleviate pain. I learned which muscles I was going to use during birth and how I was going to use them.

In a later class we became familiar with the mechanics of birth: how labor begins, the role and nature of contractions, the different phases of labor, and the birth itself. Ghislaine taught us how to respond with an effective type of breathing during each phase of labor. Finally, we learned how to aid in the expulsion of the baby.

Conscientiously we carried out the relaxation and breathing exercises. I was amazed how undemanding the practice was and how little time I had to spend— it had seemed that only great gymnastic efforts for long periods of time could achieve such results.

As we sought a Lamaze-trained doctor, Ghislaine suggested that we contact a Dr. Robert DePree, who lived in the village near us. Dr. DePree had been trained in the Lamaze technique and was interested in working with couples having their babies by this method. From the beginning we were impressed by his sincerity and enthusiasm. He treated us as if we were intelligent human beings who were interested

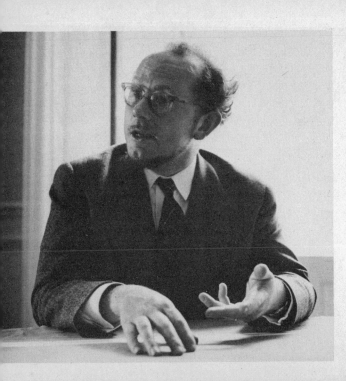

in participating in the birth of our baby. We met several times with Dr. DePree to review the knowledge we were gaining in the classes, and he concisely outlined the steps of birth—what to expect, how we were to respond, and the terminology we would use.

In the best of health and spirits, we carried on our work throughout this time. As late as the eighth month we were traveling in Spain and Portugal, continuing our photographic work. We returned to our retreat in France the last month, and began making preparations for the big day.

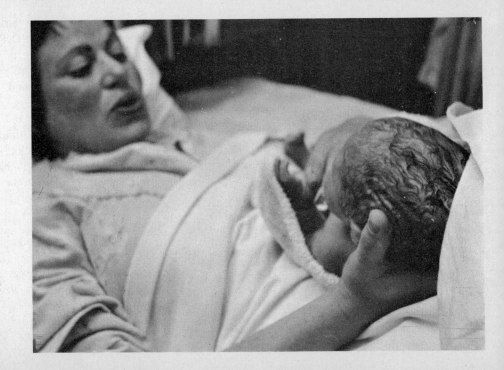

On July 18th at 3:25 A.M. our daughter Marguerite was born. During labor the techniques I had learned in the Lamaze classes proved extremely effective. They made labor a positive, controllable experience, even though it required all of my attention, concentration, and effort. When the moment of delivery finally came, we watched with amazement as the doctor delivered Marguerite's head, announcing "Here are the eyes, the nose, the mouth. *Voila,* the head is born." Another push and out came one shoulder, then the other and our baby's body eased through. We held our breaths, waiting for her cry— first a whimper and then a full, healthy wail. When Rodger laid Marguerite in my arms, we realized the fulfillment of giving birth. It was memorable to share in the birth of our child. A new child is always a work of wonder, but a mother and father participating in birth share additionally in a feeling of closeness and accomplishment.

Two years later, when our second baby was coming, we had returned to the United States. Since our experience with the first Lamaze birth, we had looked foward to finding a doctor who would be willing to deliver this next one using the same approach. Dr. Rudy DeLuise, the husband of a high-school friend, delivered our second daughter, Suzanne. Dr. DeLuise was much impressed by a prepared mother and father who were able to remain in control during labor and delivery.

When we found ourselves looking forward to the birth of our third child, Dr. DeLuise felt that Sister Margaret-Ann would be extremely interested in the use of the Lamaze technique, and invited her to participate in our birth. The birth of our son Rodger convinced Sister Margaret-Ann of the merit of preparation. She felt that the community would benefit if a Lamaze program was made available to those who were interested in receiving such preparation for child-

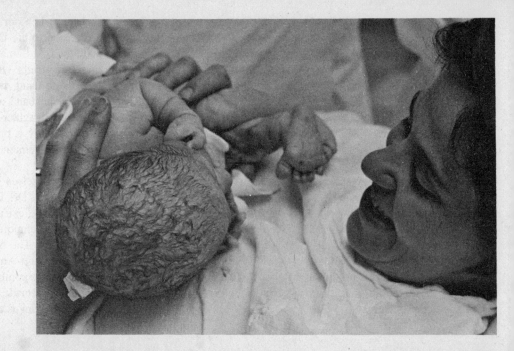

birth, and with her encouragement we began a Lamaze program at St. Anthony's Hospital. Leon, our last Lamaze baby, born two years later, completed our family.

A Denver obstetrician, Dr. Harvey Cohen, was interested in Lamaze training for his patients and contacted us. He expressed interest and enthusiasm for our program and sent patients for training. Their positive attitudes, along with their willingness and ability to cooperate with the doctor, convinced him of the benefits of preparation. Throughout the following years, Dr. Cohen has contributed his full support and enthusiasm to the Lamaze program.

This book began with the birth of our first child. Sister Margaret-Ann's "Would that more couples were able to appreciate this privilege" encouraged us to write it. The final rendition, which has undergone years of modification, refinement, and revision, is presented with gratitude for the cooperation and assistance of Dr. Cohen, the fine group of people who

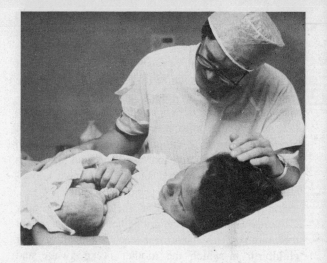

have devoted their efforts to teaching Lamaze, and the hundreds of women and their husbands who have attended our classes.

Since the inception of this book in 1961, the art of having a baby has come a long way. From the traditional view of a woman laboring alone, a passive participant in delivery, and her newborn taken to a nursery after birth, we have come into an era of established patients' rights and responsibilities in which childbirth means active participation and in which both parents are informed and able to make knowledgeable choices.

Lamaze has been a basic factor in the Family Centered Maternity Care movement that has swept the country. This movement teaches preparation for childbirth in which the mother is an awake and aware participant in the birth of her baby and the father is an essential part of the team. Today, parents may question the routine use of anesthetics and episiotomies, mothers may choose the position that is most comfortable during labor and delivery, and parents may choose where they wish to deliver the baby. Immediately following birth, parents may request skin-to-skin contact with their newborn, nursing on the delivery table, and no separation from their baby.

Thanks to the courageous efforts of many pioneers in childbirth education and obstetrics, a parent can experience a humanized birth and still be able to receive the benefits of high-risk obstetrics and neonatology should one need it.

Why Is Training Necessary?

Although childbirth is a normal and natural function of women, it is also an intense and challenging experience. A woman who undergoes labor and delivery without preparation is very likely to find it a frustrating and unsatisfactory experience.

To participate effectively and constructively in the birth of her child, the mother-to-be must be prepared for the experience before her. A positive attitude toward childbirth will be reinforced. The trained woman recognizes the birth of a child as a normal, natural phenomenon. She learns the reason for each aspect of labor and delivery and looks forward to the events that will happen. She looks forward to her child's birth with understanding and confidence.

The unprepared mother often approaches childbirth uninformed, with negative feelings. What has her mother told her about the experience of childbirth? How have her schools prepared her? What have books, movies, and television conveyed to her? If anything, she has been taught that birth is a frightening, painful experience. When the time comes for the birth of her baby she is subconsciously, if not consciously, fearful of the experience before her.

During childbirth a woman may feel helpless. She does not know what is happening to her body, let alone what to do about it. Her husband feels that the woman he loves is suffering and that he is helpless to aid her.

The normal thing for the unprepared woman to do during labor is to respond in some way to her contractions. But how? Because no one has ever told her what to do, she reacts with the most basic of responses: she tenses her whole body during each contraction. Her tensing causes the contraction to become painful and the "fear-tension-pain" cycle goes into action.

A tense, frightened woman in labor may hold her breath or perhaps overbreathe, producing an imbalance of oxygen in her system. Over a period of time she finds herself more tense, exhausted, and out of control.

To an untrained woman, the contractions usually seem to last an extremely long time. Sometimes she cannot discern their beginning or end. In a state of fear and tension, she soon becomes exhausted. When

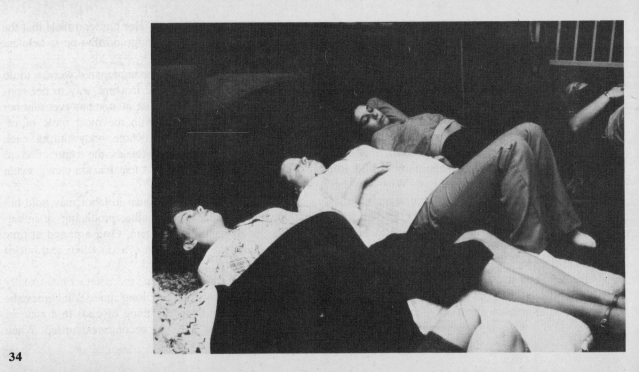

she is exhausted, any strong sensation becomes painful and difficult to control.

All of these factors—fear, ignorance, helplessness, tension, imbalance of oxygen, and exhaustion—contribute to the discomfort of a woman during labor and delivery. She feels every contraction with more intensity, fears it during its occurrence, and dreads each succeeding one. To her, each contraction is a signal for her to feel pain.

Training for Childbirth

In training, a woman not only learns what is going to happen to her during labor and delivery, but also acquires techniques that will help her control her body. Instead of tensing against the contractions of childbirth, she is prepared to consciously relax her body. She also learns to respond to each contraction with a specific type of breathing that helps her keep a normal amount of oxygen in her system and, perhaps more important, gives her a correct response to concentrate on during each contraction. She is able to analyze the beginning, apex, and end of each contraction and can take advantage of the time between contractions to replenish her reserves of energy. Her husband has been instructed how to be of utmost help at this time. To a prepared woman, a contraction is a signal to begin her work.

These elements—a positive attitude, knowledge, confidence, relaxation, breathing techniques, and the ability to conserve energy—prepare a woman to assume an active, fulfilling role in childbirth.

What Is the Lamaze Method?

Basically, the Lamaze method prepares a woman emotionally, intellectually, psychologically, and physically for childbirth. The trained woman approaches childbirth with a positive attitude. She is aware of the mechanics of labor and delivery, and she knows how to work with the functions of her body. She is psychologically prepared to respond to the challenging experience before her. And she is physically equipped with techniques for coping with the demands of childbirth.

The Lamaze method is based upon Pavlov's principle of the conditioned response, the theory that the brain can be trained to accept and analyze a given stimulus, and select a response to it.

Russian psychologists, calling their method psychoprophylaxis (or "mind-prevention"), trained pregnant women to respond positively to the uterine contractions of childbirth. They found that women who had been taught to regard birth as a positive experience and trained to respond to their uterine contractions with effective breathing and relaxation techniques could experience childbirth with a minimum of discomfort. The high activity level of these techniques, moreover, acted as a distraction that alleviated or eliminated the sensations of pain.

The Russians presented their program of psychoprophylaxis to a gynecological conference in Paris in 1950, where Dr. Lamaze, then head of an obstetrical clinic, became acquainted with the concept. Dr. Lamaze went to Russia to become more familiar with the techniques. He added the rapid accelerated breathing technique to psychoprophylaxis and set up a modified psychoprophylaxis program in France that today is known as "Accouchement sans Douleur" or "Childbirth without Pain." It is practiced throughout Europe, South America, Africa, and the United States, as well as in many eastern countries. Since Dr. Lamaze's death his protégé, Dr. Pierre Vellay, has provided leadership and guidance to the international movement.

Modification of Lamaze

As used in the United States, Lamaze has been further modified from its original concepts, especially in the use of anesthetics, the evaluation of pain, and the context of conditioning exercises.

Lamaze Is Not Childbirth without Anesthetics

Because a trained woman approaches childbirth relaxed, knowledgeable, and prepared, there is naturally less need for anesthetics. Her training will alleviate or even eliminate the need for anesthetics in a normal delivery. However, the prepared woman is also taught to realize that there is a possibility that for the safety of her baby or herself the doctor may have to intervene at any time. She is ready to give her fullest cooperation and support to the medical staff working with her. Her primary concern is to deliver a healthy baby; of secondary importance is how she delivers it.

Lamaze Is Not Childbirth without Pain

Although some women do experience childbirth without pain, there are certain physical factors in birth that may cause real pain regardless of training. The physical structure of the woman, the size of her baby, the quality of contractions, and complications of labor are but a few of the real physical problems that may contribute to pain. Although training tends to alleviate the pain factor, the aim of training is not to make childbirth painless but to make it a controllable, positive experience. Even if pain is present, the prepared mother regards her labor and delivery as a time of activity, work, concentration and confidence, rather than a time of passiveness, helplessness, anguish, or suffering.

Lamaze Is Not "Natural Childbirth"

Although the Dick-Read method of natural childbirth was one of the first to recognize the importance of a woman's positive attitude in childbirth, it stopped at the philosophical implications of birth. "Natural childbirth" is based upon positive thinking, passive relaxation, and a touch of mysticism. A great deal of emphasis is placed upon the woman's "performance." The Lamaze method, on the contrary, is founded on sound scientific principles. It is based upon scientifically devised means of dealing with contractions. The woman is conditioned to respond to contractions with "unnatural"—and effective—responses. Proponents of the Lamaze method advocate the use of anesthetics and obstetrical techniques when required. Emphasis is placed upon the woman's attitude rather than upon her performance.

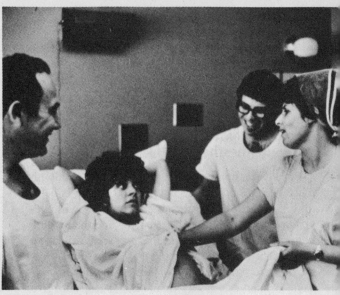

Advantages of Lamaze

Probably the greatest advantage of the Lamaze technique is that it allows the woman to assume an active role in one of the most creative events in her life. She approaches childbirth with confidence and knowledge, and she is able to maintain control and dignity throughout her labor. As a participant in the drama of her child's birth, she experiences childbirth as a dignified and fulfilling experience.

The father who participates enjoys a unique and beautiful experience—being actively involved in the birth of his child. He is part of the team and is not banished as a germ-ridden foreign object to the father's room. Sharing this experience with his wife promotes mutual closeness and appreciation.

The few hours spent in childbirth will be among the most profound and real hours spent in your life. Childbirth is often the first meaningful challenge a young couple has to face. If the experience of childbirth is met with control and dignity, the husband and wife emerge with new confidence.

Many options have been expressed on the advantages for the baby of a prepared birth. Certainly there is an advantage in minimizing the use of drugs; however, probably the greatest advantage is that the baby is born into an environment where harmony and cooperation prevail.

The function of Lamaze education is to provide preparation for childbirth as a link between the mother, father, doctor, and attending nurse. The doctor and the medical staff enjoy working with a woman who is knowledgeable and who is able to participate and cooperate intelligently with them. They are able to communicate and work together to achieve a safe, happy delivery and a healthy baby.

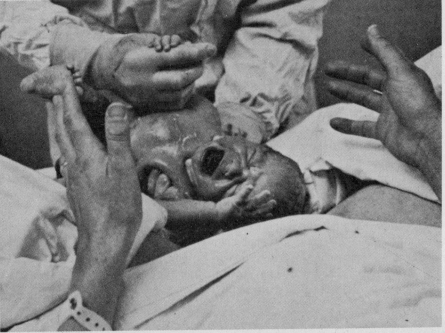

Preparation for Childbirth

The following chapters are devoted to preparing you for childbirth. They describe in detail the anatomy of birth, the mechanisms of labor and delivery, techniques for muscular control, breathing techniques, and, finally, the birth.

The techniques you will acquire through these lessons will equip you to work *with* your labor. They will be your response to the demanding experience of childbirth.

The easier your labor, of course, the easier your task. Just as some women are pretty or intelligent, some have easy labors. If you are lucky you may have a short, easy, "normal" labor. If, however, you are not so favored, you may have a long, hard, complicated labor. You bear no responsibility for the type of labor you chance to have. Be prepared to approach your labor with determination and

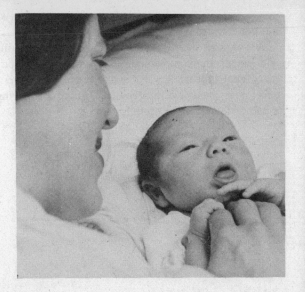

preseverance, as you would any challenging task, but don't try to be a martyr or a hero.

A prepared mother and modern obstetrical skills and anesthetic complement each other. Your primary goal is a healthy baby and a positive experience; how you deliver is secondary. Success is having a baby—there can be no failure.

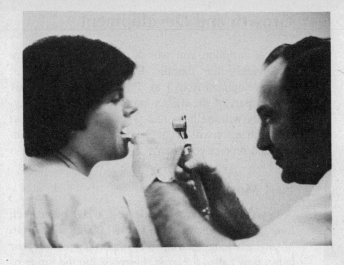

Chapter Two:
A Healthy Pregnancy

Introduction

The greatest gift you can give your baby during pregnancy is a healthy beginning to life. In fact, what you do during pregnancy affects not only the baby's development but its health for the rest of its life.

Your gifts include: early prenatal care, understanding of your baby's development during pregnancy, knowledge about the changes in your body during pregnancy, good nutrition, plenty of rest and relaxation, good daily care, and early planning to ensure family-centered maternity care throughout your pregnancy and childbirth experiences.

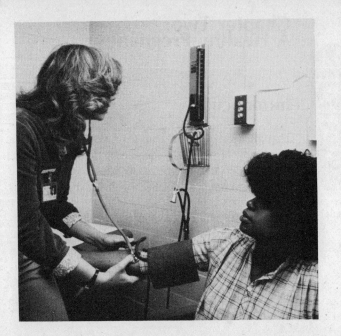

Growth and Development

After conception you will nurture the baby for approximately nine months. During this time, his or her development from 1 to 200 billion cells will only be one part of the miraculous drama of pregnancy. Not only will the baby and your abdomen grow, but many changes will occur inside your body to maintain and protect your baby.

First Month

Your Baby: From a single cell 1/200 of an inch long, the baby increases in size 10,000 times to 1/16 of an inch long. During this important month your baby, now called a *zygote,* burrows into the lining of the uterus and the formation of the placenta and umbilical cord begins. The cells of the fertilized egg arrange themselves into three layers, in preparation for the development of the major organs. The beginnings of the brain, spine, and vital organs are evident.

Your Body: You may experience nausea or morning sickness and you may have to urinate frequently. Perhaps you will feel a sensation of swelling and tenderness in your breasts. Your temperature rises and you may miss your menstrual period for the first time.

Second Month

Your Baby: By the second month your baby is called an *embryo*. The heart begins to beat and circulate blood. Arm and leg buds emerge and the backbone, brain, spinal cord, and nervous system are established. The digestive system forms and arms and legs begin to grow. The umbilical cord joins the embryo to the placenta and the long bones and internal organs are developing. Your baby grows from 1/6 of an inch long to 1/2 an inch long and now weighs 1/30 of an ounce.

Your Body: During the second month your breasts enlarge and are tender. You may experience irregular uterine contractions and notice changes in the senses of taste and smell or crave certain kinds of food.

Third Month

Your Baby: The baby is now called a *fetus* and resembles a human. Its face, arms, legs, fingers, toes, elbows, knees, eyelids, and bone cells are forming. During the third month sex is distinguishable and fingers and toes are moving. Teeth buds are present. The fetus has grown from 1/2 inch long and 1/30 of an ounce to 1 and 3/4 inches long and a weight of 1 ounce.

Your Body: During the third month you may notice colostrum, a yellowish sticky fluid, seeping from your breasts. Your blood supply increases to provide needed nutrients to the fetus. Your center of gravity shifts. Nausea usually begins to subside.

Fourth Month

Your Baby: A baby moves and kicks, sleeps and wakes. Hair begins to form and skin is pink in color. Your baby swallows amniotic fluid.

Your Body: In the fourth month you begin to gain weight and to notice your abdomen enlarging. You may experience a new sense of physical well being. Increase in hormones may cause heartburn and a darker skin pigmentation on your face, breasts, and abdomen.

Fifth Month

Your Baby: During the fifth month a baby experiences a spurt in growth. It is now 8–12 inches long and weighs up to 3/4 of a pound. The face is red and wrinkled and eyebrows and lashes can be seen. Eyelids can open and close. Your baby is now storing large amounts of iron. Its skin is covered with a cheeselike protective coating called vernix.

Your Body: A very important thing happens during the fifth month. You begin to feel the baby move and feel life within you. As the uterus expands to the level of your navel, abdominal skin stretches and you may feel increased pressure on your rectum. Hormones may cause relaxation of your smooth muscles, resulting in constipation, varicose veins, or hemorrhoids.

Sixth Month

Your Baby: By now a baby weighs 1 and 3/4 pounds and is 11–14 inches long. The outline of the fetus can be felt from your abdomen. Its skin is red and shiny, and the face is wrinkled.

Your Body: The sixth month is the one in which the greatest weight gain occurs. You can feel the vigorous movements of your baby. Hormones cause heavy pigmentation of your body, resulting in the mask of pregnancy and *linea nigra* (a dark line that extends from pubic hair to navel). Hormones cause ligaments to stretch and your iron level begins to drop.

Seventh Month

Your Baby: The seventh month is the period of the most rapid growth for your baby. It is now 15 inches long and weighs 2½–3 pounds. The central nervous system is developed enough so that if a baby were born now, it could survive with special care. Eyelids can open and close. The body is filling out and internal organs are almost completely formed.

Your Body: The growing weight of a baby causes increased stress on all of your body's systems. Both the structural and hormonal changes can cause backaches, muscle strain, increased nasal congestion and nosebleeds, and stretch marks. Braxton-Hicks (or early) contractions may be felt. Blood volume increases.

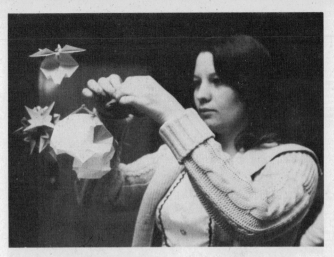

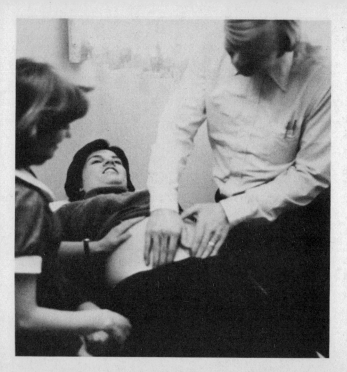

Eighth Month

Your Baby: The baby grows to 16–18 inches long and weighs 4–5 pounds. It now settles into a favorite position and valuable fat deposits increase. All systems have matured and a fetus can survive birth.

Your Body: Heavy demands for calcium and iron are being made on your body. You feel strong movements from the baby and experience stronger contractions. Colostrum secretions are increasing. Increased weight gain and hormones may cause muscle cramps, stretch marks, and muscle spasms.

Ninth Month

Your Baby: A baby now gains 1/2 pound per week. It is about 18 inches long and weighs 7–8 pounds. The bones of the head are soft and flexible and internal organs are well developed. The respiratory system is mature. Fingernails reach fingertips. As your baby accumulates fat, its skin smooths out and becomes pink.

Family-Centered Maternity Care

Early and good prenatal care begins, if possible, even before your baby is conceived and born. General maternal health affects a developing fetus even before pregnancy. From the moment you first suspect you are pregnant, contact your doctor, clinic, or certified midwife and make an appointment for your first visit.

Whom you choose to surround yourself with and give you medical care during your pregnancy and childbirth will be among the most important choices of your life. Take time to develop a philosophy about what you want from this experience. Explore sources of information concerning alternatives and choices offered in pregnancy and childbirth. A healthy and happy baby, mother, and family is your most important goal. How you go about achieving this goal is very important. Your medical caregiver—whether obstetrician, family practitioner, certified midwife, or clinic attendant—will help you attain the experiences you want.

The experiences you have during your pregnancy, childbirth, and the early days following birth have a great effect on how you will parent your newborn. People who provide family-centered maternity care are concerned about you as a family. They provide an atmosphere and facilities that foster the development of warm and loving feelings between the family and the newborn. When you choose your medical caregiver and the facility where you wish to give birth, choose those that will provide the following:

1. Preparation for the mother and the father that will help you both become informed and active participants in the birth of your baby.

49

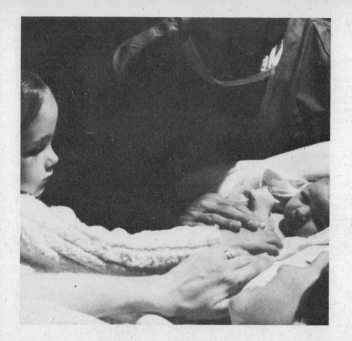

2. A medical team which supports you as a family and gives you the information, confidence, and support you need.

3. A range of choices and alternatives such as the father being allowed in the delivery room, delivery in the labor room, birthing rooms, early breastfeeding.

4. A view of the birth process as a normal, natural phenomenon that is not only the birth of a baby, but the birth of a family.

5. Respect for the comfort and dignity of the mother, baby, and father during labor and delivery.

6. A minimal use of medical and obstetrical intervention; no routine use of anesthesia, medications, IV's, episiotomies, or inductions of labor.

7. Understanding of the significance of family bonding during the early hours following delivery and appreciation of this as a special time for baby, mother, and father to remain together as a family unit.

Nutrition

Good nutrition is especially important to you and your growing baby. Research shows that good nutrition can reduce your chances of having problems during pregnancy and complications during labor and delivery. Good nutrition helps prevent premature birth and increases the probability of having a healthy, normal-size baby.

The food that you ingest contains the only nutrients that your baby will receive. A balanced diet gives a baby an early start to good health. Provide your body with the proteins, carbohydrates, fats, vitamins, and minerals the baby needs for growth and development.

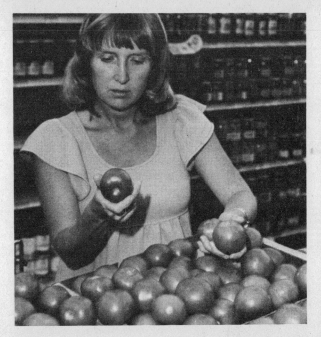

Nutrients: Protein, Carbohydrates, Fats, Vitamins, and Minerals

Your baby needs proteins as basic building materials for his or her growth and development. Protein is vital for brain and cell growth during gestation. A fetus needs carbohydrates for brain and cell growth and development. It must be provided with fats for brain development and body temperature regulation. Vitamin A encourages healthy development of skeleton, skin, hair, gums, glands, and teeth enamel. Development of the baby's nervous system is promoted by the complex of B vitamins. Vitamin C is essential for your baby's teeth and bone development, and Vitamin D is also needed to build strong teeth and bones.

An increased intake of calcium, iron, and folic acid is essential in building teeth and bones and is important for the normal growth and development of your baby's body cells.

Basic Food Groups

You can supply these nutrients by being sure you get the following foods daily:

Dairy Products: the equivalent of one quart of Vitamin D fortified milk, such as whole or skim milk, yogurt, buttermilk, or cheese

Protein: two generous servings of meat, fish, poultry, eggs, nuts, dry beans, peas, or lentils

Vegetables: two large portions of dark green, leafy or other green vegetable

Fruit: one food high in Vitamin C such as citrus fruit, berries, melon, peppers, tomatoes, or cabbage

Cereal: four servings of whole-grain cereal or bread

Other: at least one more serving of any fruit, vegetable, or potato

Water: 6–8 glasses

Eat foods that are healthful and concentrate on

getting enough protein. Be sure to eat those that are especially rich in vitamins and minerals. Avoid foods that contain many calories and few nutrients; make a conscientious effort to avoid junk foods.

Weight Gain

One of the first concerns is how much weight you should gain. Weight gain is the result of both the growth of your baby and the changes in your body. The baby grows to add approximately 8 pounds to your total weight; the placenta 1 pound; and the amniotic fluid 2 more. Your breasts each enlarge about 1 pound and your uterus 2 pounds. The increase in your blood volume adds 3 more pounds. Fat stored in the abdominal wall, back, thighs, and breasts to provide a ready source of energy for the growth of your baby adds another 6 pounds, totalling a *minimum* weight gain of 24 pounds.

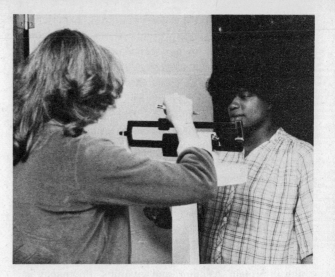

During the first trimester, you may experience only a slight increase in weight. About half of your weight gain occurs in the second trimester and another half in the last trimester. Although there are wide variations, you probably gain 25 percent of your normal weight during your pregnancy; that is, 110–138 pounds, 120–150 pounds, or 130–163 pounds.

Non-pregnant women of childbearing age need approximately 2100 calories daily to provide enough energy for good health and ordinary activity. During pregnancy, you need not only increase your daily caloric intake to 2400 but make every calorie count by planning a diet based on nutrient-rich foods.

If you are overweight at the beginning of your pregnancy, be sure to cut back on high-caloric foods, empty of nutrients, rather than eliminating foods high in protein, calcium, and vitamins. Pregnancy is not the time to try to lose weight. Recent evidence shows that a baby's brain grows most rapidly during the last two months of pregnancy. A low-calorie, low-protein diet may actually harm fetal brain development.

Rest and Relaxation

Stress during your pregnancy can affect both you and your baby. It is associated with complications during pregnancy, childbirth, and postpartum. Try to avoid stressful situations and to surround yourself with people and experiences that bring you peace.

Five minutes of relaxation can be like a half-hour of sleep. Every day, as a minimum, take out 5–15 minutes for relaxation. First, get into comfortable clothing, empty your bladder, darken the room, take the phone off the hook, and either slip into bed or find a comfortable place where you can completely relax. Tell yourself that this is the time for you and your baby. Get into a comfortable position by supporting your body with pillows under your head, legs, and arms. Close your eyes and think about each part of your body.

Concentrate on letting the tension flow out. As you breathe in, think of breathing in warm relaxing air; as you breathe out, think of breathing out all of the tension in your body. Relax your face and let your jaw drop. Relax your neck and chest. Concentrate on feeling the tension drain out. Let your breathing be even, natural, and effortless. Relax the muscles of your abdomen. Relax your legs and thighs; feel how your thighs become heavy and loose. Relax your feet, letting them fall naturally from your body. Concentrate on feeling the tension flow out of your body. Feel the support of your pillows. Focus on the heaviness and limpness of your body when it is totally relaxed. Imagine you are lying in the middle of a beautiful scene that is absolutely at peace: at the seaside, in a meadow, or in the mountains.

Take a moment to create a scene around you that is peaceful and relaxing: the warm sun, a light breeze, clouds drifting by in the sky, etc. Then, take in five deep breaths, and with each breath imagine that you are even more relaxed. Sink deeper and deeper and feel your body become heavier and heavier. Enjoy the feeling. Take several minutes to appreciate your vacation spot. Concentrate on the feeling of complete peace and relaxation. When you feel you are ready, slowly begin to move, roll over to your side, and push yourself up.

Take time out each day for relaxation. As your pregnancy progresses, increase your relaxation sessions to two or three times a day.

Body-Building Exercises

The following body-building exercises are designed to build up muscle support during pregnancy and labor, contribute to more effective pushing during delivery, and provide good muscle tone after the birth of your baby.

These are not the "end-all" for prenatal exercises. You can obtain many other excellent groups of exercises from other books on pregnancy and from your doctor.

Practice each exercise three times each for two daily sessions, perhaps one in the morning and one in the evening.

Posture

Good posture cannot be emphasized enough. It relieves backaches and makes you feel and look better.

Tuck in buttocks, tilt pelvis forward to align spine, shoulders gently back, arms relaxed, head erect, and chin in.

Practice: at all times.

56

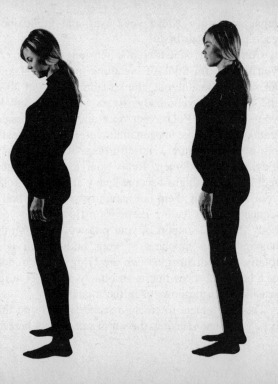

Pelvic-Floor Muscles

Good all around exercise.

Position: lie on back, legs straight, crossed at ankles.

Contract buttocks and hold. Still contracting buttocks, squeeze legs together and contract thigh muscles and hold. Next, contract pelvic-floor muscles (uretha, vagina, and rectum). Hold all muscles contracted and then release.

Practice: ten times twice daily

Kegal Exercise. Excellent for strengthening vaginal muscles.

Position: standing, sitting, or lying down.

Push as if urinating and then contract muscles as if to stop the flow. If it is hard to get the "feeling" of this exercise, do it when you are actually urinating. Release the urine, then contract to stop the flow. Hold for a second and repeat.

Practice: 60–100 times twice daily

Elevator Exercise: Another way to strengthen the vaginal muscles is to think of the vagina as an elevator shaft that starts at the ground and rises to the fifth floor.

Slowly begin to contract the vaginal muscles, bring them up slowly, from the first up to the second, third, fourth, and fifth floors. Hold a few seconds, then gradually begin to release from the fifth to the fourth, third, second, and first floors; then give an extra push down to the basement. This will give you a feeling of the area you will be pushing during the expulsion. Then contract the muscles back up to first floor.

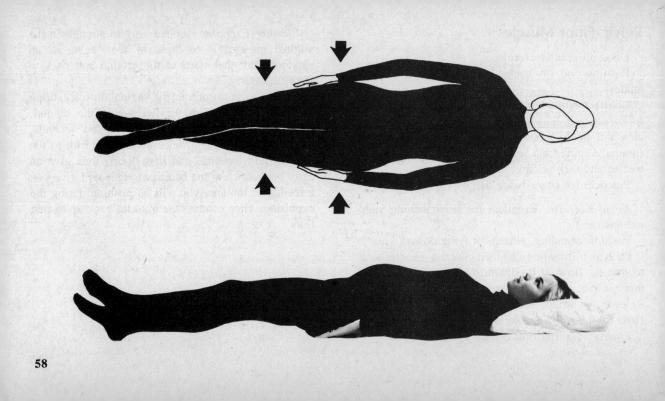

Abdominal Muscles

"Pelvic Rock." Very good for aching backs. Position: lie on back, legs bent, feet flat on floor.

Imagine your hips as a swivel point. Contract buttocks, flatten back firmly against floor, and tip pelvis forward by contracting abdominal muscles. Release. Rock pelvis three times. Repeat exercise.

Practice: ten times twice daily

Variation. Standing up. Place hands under table top, stand in a normal position with feet flat on floor. Rise onto tiptoes, drop shoulders, tuck in buttocks, tilt pelvis up, and pull up gently on the table. Release.

Practice: ten times twice daily

Variation. Lie on back, legs bent, feet flat on floor. Contract buttocks, flatten back firmly against floor, and tilt the pelvis forward. Now hold the pelvis tilted forward and slowly lift and straighten one leg. Lower your leg slowly to the floor, keeping

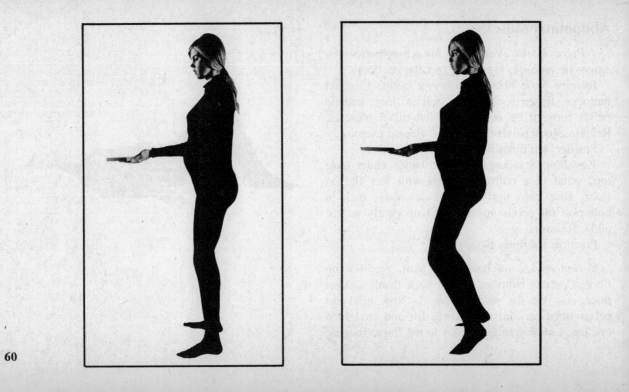

your knee straight; then return to relaxed position with knees bent. Repeat with other leg.

Practice: ten times twice daily.

Variation: On hands and knees. Start with head up, back sunken in by letting stomach sink toward the floor. Contract buttocks, pull pelvis forward, straighten back, tuck chin in. Release

Practice: ten times twice daily.

"Blowing out the Candle." Very good for strengthening abdominal muscles.

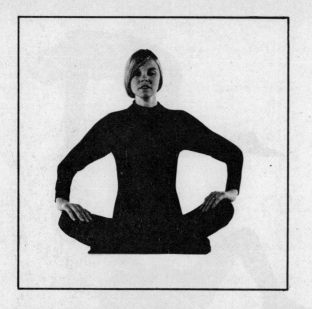

Position: lie on back, pillow under head, legs bent, feet flat on floor.

Imagine there is a burning candle about 12 inches from your lips. Take in a deep breath and let it out naturally. Now, without taking another breath, purse your lips and continue blowing as if to extinguish the flame on the candle. Keep blowing until you feel as if there is no more air and then blow some more. You will begin to feel the abdominal muscles contracting. Release.

Practice: ten times twice daily.

Stretching Exercises

Sitting Tailor Fashion

Position: sit on floor, feet crossed at ankles. Place your hands on the outside of your knees and push upward. Release inner thighs as you slowly press your knees outward.

Practice: ten times twice daily

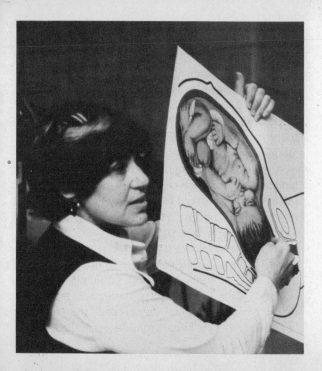

Chapter Three:
Labor and Delivery

Reproductive Organs

Preparation for childbirth is based upon understanding and knowledge. The untrained woman approaches childbirth with little or no understanding of her body and how it functions, but you will have this knowledge.

The passageway consists of the organs and structures within a woman's body through which the baby will travel in childbirth. Normal labor takes the baby on a journey through that passageway from the uterus, through the pelvis, cervix, vagina, pelvic floor, and vulva to the outside world.

What are the organs and skeletal structure that are concerned in your pregnancy, labor, and delivery?

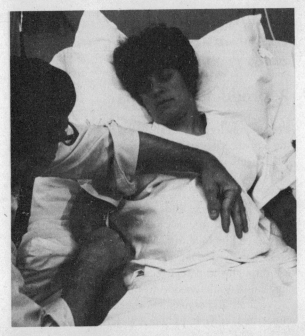

First, consider the area in the pelvic basin. Put your hands high on your hips and draw them together down low in front to the *pubic arch,* that bony hump in the middle. Now put your hands on your hips again and draw them to the back and down, as far as they will go. This is your *coccyx,* or "tailbone." This entire area is called the *pelvic basin,* and essentially it is where all the activity of your pregnancy, labor, and delivery takes place.

At birth, a baby must pass through three major landmarks in the pelvis. First, it must pass into the *inlet,* which is marked by the *pubic bone* at the front of the pelvis, the *sacrum,* or base of the spine, and the inner ridges of the hipbone.

Then it passes through the pelvic passageway measured by the *diagonal conjugate* from the bottom of the pubic bone to the top of the sacrum.

Third, your baby must pass through the *outlet,* which is marked by the pubic bone, the *coccyx* or tailbone, and two bony prominences called the *is-*

chial spines. Both inlet and outlet are oval shaped. They differ in one way: the inlet is wider from side to side and the outlet is wider from front to back.

Descent of the baby is described in stations. An imaginary line drawn across the ischial spines is called *station zero*. When your baby's head enters the inlet, it is said to be at station minus five. As its head descends into the pelvis and reaches the ischial spines at station zero, it is said to be *engaged*. When the head passes this critical landmark it indicates that the measurements of the mother's pelvis are adequate for the birth of her baby.

Within the pelvic basin are the organs that are responsible for the conception and growth of the baby within you now. The main organ is the *uterus* (see Diagram), which is a hollow, thick-walled muscle. Extending from both sides of the uterus, near the top, are the *Fallopian tubes*. At the ends of the tubes and somewhat tucked under them are two small, almond-shaped organs called the *ovaries*. During the

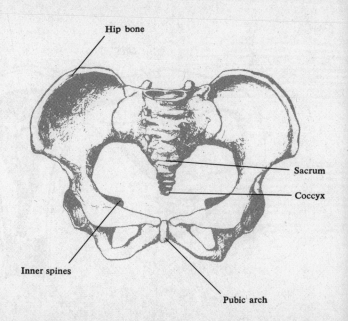

Hip bone

Sacrum

Coccyx

Inner spines

Pubic arch

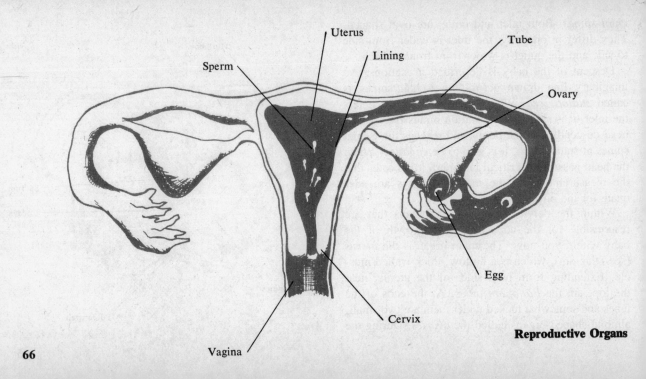

Uterus

Lining

Sperm

Tube

Ovary

Egg

Cervix

Vagina

Reproductive Organs

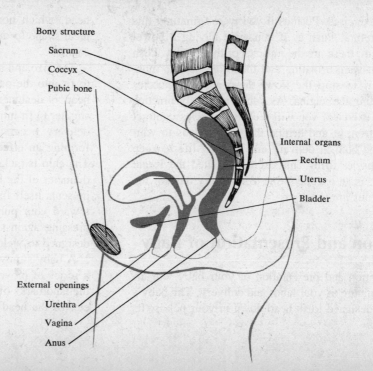

Pelvis (Cross-Section)

Bony structure

Sacrum

Coccyx

Pubic bone

Internal organs

Rectum

Uterus

Bladder

External openings

Urethra

Vagina

Anus

69

lowing exercises. Push as if you were urinating: this is the urethra. Push as if you were having a bowel movement: these are the muscles of the rectum. Push as if you were urinating and then contract the muscles as if to stop the flow: these are the muscles surrounding the vagina. As you consciously practice this last exercise, you will feel the muscles contract both in front of and behind the vagina. It is to your advantage both in delivery and in daily life to keep these muscles firm. This exercise, called the Kegal exercise, is an excellent one to do every day for the rest of your life.

Position and Presentation of Baby

The position and presentation of your baby will affect the nature of your labor and delivery. The baby's body is designed to fit head down in your pelvis. Its head, which normally emerges first in birth, is an ideal shape to dilate, or stretch, the cervix and birth canal.

The size and shape of the head and body are made to fit into the pelvis, which is flexible. Your baby's head is designed in sections and thus can become smaller to fit into your pelvis. An optimum labor and delivery occurs when the head points downward, forming an effective wedge for opening the cervix. The chin is tucked into the chest so that the smallest diameter of the back of the head, called the *occiput*, presents itself first. With the back of its head turned toward your pubic bone, the soft part of its face is pressing against the tailbone, which is flexible and designed to yield to pressure.

A baby's movements also facilitate birth. Through a series of movements, the baby maneuvers through the landmarks of your pelvis, matching largest diameter of the head measurement to largest diameter of the pelvic measurement, much like turning a foot into a tight-fitting boot. Your baby will turn its head sideways to fit the shape of your pelvic inlet, which is normally widest from side to side. Because a baby's head is widest from front to back, it usually enters the pelvis facing toward your right or left side. The outlet of a woman's pelvis is widest from front to back, so as the baby descends its head adapts by turning toward your back. As the nape of its neck passes under your pubic bone, the head gradually lifts from its chest, the neck extends and the largest part of the head emerges. This process is the *crowning*. Your baby is usually born head facing down toward your back. After the head emerges, it automatically rotates back to the side to align with the shoulders, which are still sideways in your pelvis. The baby's passage through the tight birth canal has put pressure on its chest, which helps express mucus from his lungs.

Contractions

Probably one of the greatest fears a woman has concerning childbirth is how can a baby pass through such an obviously small opening without excruciating pain. The whole function of "labor" is to allow the contractions of the uterus to open the cervix (the lower part of the uterus) to about 4 inches, the diameter of the baby's head. After the cervix has opened, the baby passes through the birth canal.

Contractions are the means by which labor and delivery take place. The better you understand the nature and role of your contractions, the better you can cope with them during labor. An untrained woman going into labor usually interprets her contractions as "pains." To her a contraction is only the signal for another oncoming pain to be endured. An educated woman learns that contractions are the mechanism by which the cervix is opened and her baby expelled. She looks forward to each contraction as a step further in the progress of the birth of her baby. The contraction is her signal to begin relaxation, controlled breathing, and concentration on a focal point. The contraction is the coach's signal to begin massage and to give guidance and encouragement.

What is a contraction? The uterus is a set of muscles, just like the muscles in your arm. There is one great difference, however; the muscles in your arm are voluntary muscles and the muscles of the uterus are involuntary. They contract whether you want them to or not. Once in labor, you can't decide to come back later. By pulling up (or contracting), the muscles of the uterus open up the cervix and expel the baby.

To understand the nature of your contractions, it is most helpful to analyze the contractions that take place during your eighth and ninth month of pregnancy. These preliminary contractions are called Braxton-Hicks contractions after the man who formally described them in medical literature. Although they are quite different in nature from those you will experience during labor, they will help you to become familiar with the nature and sensation of the "real thing."

Place your hand on the top of your abdomen just as a contraction is starting. You will feel a slight hardening, or tightening, of the muscles, starting above the pubis, spreading toward the groin, and covering the whole uterus. The uterus will become quite hard, remain tight for a few moments, then progressively become softer until it returns to its normal state. This may take, in all, from 30 to 60 seconds. During labor, your contractions will be similar, but with three great differences: they will be stronger in intensity, longer in duration, and regular in occurrence.

The increasing and decreasing of the contractions

are similar to the mounting and subsiding of a wave. It starts slowly, increases in intensity, reaches a crest, and then subsides. During labor it may be helpful to picture a contraction as an ocean wave—you can see it gathering, breaking, and subsiding. If you have ever gone swimming in the ocean surf, you know that if you stand up to a wave and fight it you will be knocked down and pulled under. However, if you lie down in the water and work with the wave you will be able to control it. The wave and the contraction are powerful elements. The best way to control them is to work with, not against, them.

During the first part of the contraction you can use your breathing and relaxation techniques easily. When the contraction reaches its apex, you must work hard to maintain control. As the contraction subsides, you can easily maintain control. Since the entire contraction lasts only about 60 seconds and the apex only a few seconds, you will usually have only 20 to 30 seconds of really hard work for each contraction, and you get from 1 to 5 minutes of rest between contractions.

Labor and Delivery

Your physician may talk about three phases of labor. The first includes *effacement, dilatation,* and *transition.* The second phase is *expulsion,* and the third phase is delivery of the placenta. Simplified for our purpose, labor and delivery will be divided into four stages: effacement, dilatation, transition, and expulsion. The delivery of the placenta, or afterbirth, needs little response on your part and so we will consider it separately.

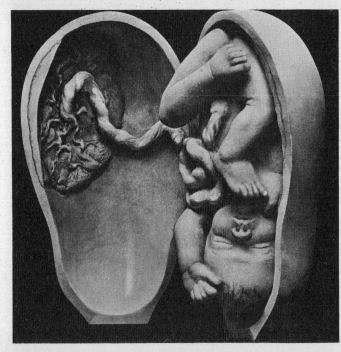

Full term baby, positioned head down, ready for birth

Photos on pages 74–80 reproduced with permission from the Birth Atlas, published by Maternity Center Association, New York.

Effacement

The foremost consideration in labor is the enlarging of the opening (cervix) to a diameter through which your baby's head can pass. During birth the normal presentation of the baby is with his head at the bottom of the uterus. The cervix makes up the passageway from the uterus to the birth canal, and can be considered as a narrow, tubular channel. The walls are made of thick elastic tissue that must be thinned out (or effaced) before the cervix can start its function of opening wider. Your labor will start so gradually that you probably will not even be aware of it at first. The contractions, which at this phase are working to efface the cervix, are relatively weak and last from 30 to 60 seconds, with regular intervals of from 5 to 20 minutes between them.

When you are first examined in the hospital you will hear much discussion about the effacement of the cervix. Your first efforts of labor are concen-

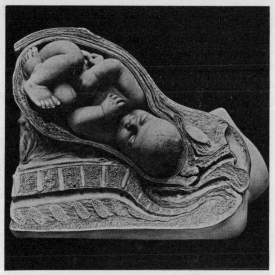

Uneffaced cervix

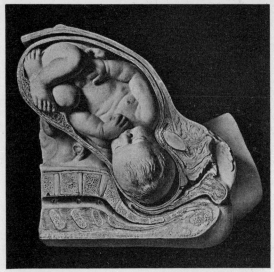

Full effaced cervix

trated on thinning the cervix and incorporating it into the walls of the uterus. The doctor or nurse will examine the cervix through the vagina where the progress of the contractions may be ascertained.

Dilatation

When the cervix has been completely thinned out and incorporated into the uterus, you will then progress into the next phase of labor, *dilatation*. Dilatation means opening up, and the contractions during dilatation concentrate their efforts on widening the diameter of the cervix so that the baby's head may pass into the birth canal. The latter part of effacement may take place with the beginning of dilatation. With each succeeding contraction, the cervix is opened slightly more. During the first phase of dilatation you will find your contractions becoming increasingly stronger, lasting for approximately 1 minute with rest intervals of 1 to 3 minutes.

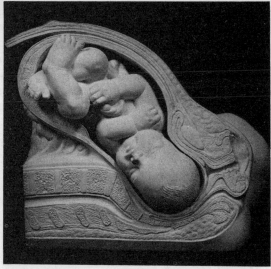

Cervix dilated 4–5 centimetres

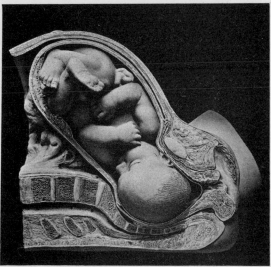

Cervix completely dilated

You will hear the nurses and your doctor speak in terms of centimetres. When the cervix is opened to the extent of about the end of your little finger, it will be opened 1 centimetre. When the opening is big enough for the baby's head to pass through, it is 10 centimetres (or about 4 inches) in diameter. This is full dilatation, or, as the French call it, "une grande pomme"—a large apple!

Transition

Transition is marked by the baby's descent into the pelvic basin, so that you feel pressure on the pelvic floor.

Just when you have become accustomed to the nature of your contractions, usually somewhere around 7 centimetres, you will become aware of a change in their quality. It will be hard to describe, but you will feel that, in addition to becoming longer and strong-er, the contractions are changing in their nature. This is because, although you are not yet fully dilated, the expulsive efforts of the uterus are beginning to exert their influence. The contractions become, for a relatively short time, quite intense. They can last anywhere from 1 to 2 minutes and are close together, with little rest in between. *You must concentrate very hard to control your response to these contractions*. However, it helps to remember that the transition usually lasts only a very short time, sometimes as little as 5 to 10 minutes.

When the cervix has been completely dilated (10 centimetres), the contractions feel less strong and seem to last a shorter time. Above all, you find yourself at last ready to give birth to your baby.

Expulsion

Finally the cervix is opened, the baby has descended into the birth canal, and all that remains is the expulsion. This final stage requires the greatest effort but also yields the greatest sense of accomplishment. The strength of the contractions reverts to about the same intensity as during dilatation. They vary in length, being usually about 60 seconds, and you will again have 1 to 3 minutes between them.

As the baby descends through the birth canal, his head rests on the floor of the pelvic region. The first expelling efforts push the head under the pubic bone. Additional pushes produce the crowning of the baby's head, where you can see your baby—about 2 inches of the top of his head. The succeeding pushes produce first his eyes, then his nose, mouth, chin—and his head is born! Another push and his shoulder appears, and then his other shoulder, and his little body comes right out. Your baby is born! The umbilical cord is cut, but your work is not over. As everyone is admiring your baby (and seems to forget about you), you will feel another contraction come on. This is the contraction of the uterus that expels

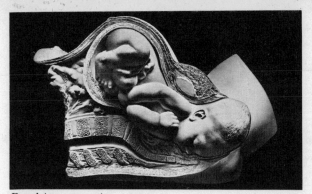
Expulsion—crowning

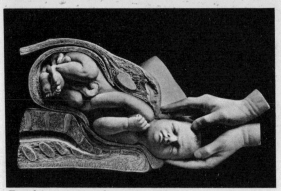

Expulsion—external rotation of head

the afterbirth, or placenta, the last stage of birth. Usually the doctor will ask you to push, and he will help you to expel the placenta.

Every woman wants to know "How long will my labor last?" and "How long does it take to deliver my baby?" All we can answer is that it is impossible to predict. Each woman and each pregnancy is different. The "normal" labor lasts usually about 8 to 12 hours, perhaps less for the woman who has had other babies (4 to 9 hours), and sometimes more for the woman who is having her first baby. The expulsion takes anywhere from half an hour to 2 hours.

There are two important facts to remember. First, labor is a series of contractions. Each contraction starts slowly, builds up, and lets off. There is an interval between contractions, so even though labor may last 12 hours, you are really working only 3 to 4 hours of this time. Second, although your labor may last 12 hours, it is actually the effacement and dilatation that takes the longest time; transition and

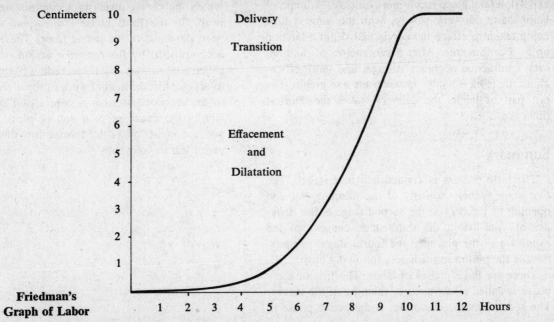

Centimeters 10 — Delivery

9

Transition

8

7

6

5 — Effacement

4 — and

3 — Dilatation

2

1

**Friedman's
Graph of Labor**

1 2 3 4 5 6 7 8 9 10 11 12 Hours

expulsion take place much more quickly. A graph of labor starts out very slowly, with the longest time being taken to efface the cervix and begin dilatation up to 5 centimetres. After 5 centimetres of dilation, each contraction becomes stronger and more efficacious; there is a sharp upsweep on our graph. The last part of labor, the delivery, takes the shortest time.

Summary

The birth process is divided into four stages. The first stage, *labor,* consists of the thinning out and opening of the cervix; the second stage is the *delivery* of your baby; the third stage consists of the *expulsion* of the placenta; the fourth stage, *postpartum,* is the period immediately following birth.

There are three phases of labor. The first or early phase is called *effacement,* or thinning of the cervix. The second phase, *dilatation,* is the active phase in which the cervix opens to accommodate the baby's head. In the third phase, *transition,* your baby's head descends to the pelvic floor. These phases are accomplished by the muscular action of the uterus, called contractions. Each succeeding contraction helps to accomplish the natural work of the uterus. Whereas to an untrained woman a contraction seems to be simply the cause of pain and helpless anguish, to you a contraction is the mechanism that helps you give birth to your baby.

Outline of Contractions

Early (Effacement)

Purpose	To soften, thin out, and partially open the cervix
Intensity	Variable; usually light, easy to control
Length	From 30 to 60 seconds
Interval	From 5 to 20 minutes
Duration	Varies greatly with each individual

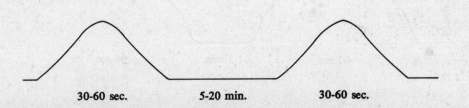

30-60 sec.   5-20 min.   30-60 sec.

Active (Dilatation)

Purpose	To open the cervix from 3 to approximately 7 centimetres
Intensity	Stronger and harder to manage, but controllable
Length	60 seconds
Interval	From 1 to 3 minutes
Duration	First baby, 5 to 9 hours; other children, 2 to 5 hours

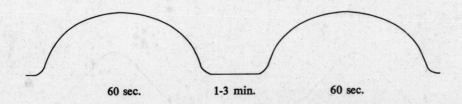

60 sec.   1-3 min.   60 sec.

Transition

Purpose	Continuing to open the cervix (from 7 to 10 centimetres), and pushing the baby down into the birth canal
Intensity	Extremely strong and erratic; more difficult to manage
Length	From 60 to 90 seconds
Interval	About 1 minute; may be erratic
Duration	Usually short

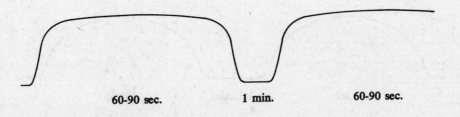

60-90 sec.   1 min.   60-90 sec.

Expulsion

Purpose	To expel the baby from the uterus
Intensity	Less strong than during the transitional stage; controllable
Length	About 60 seconds (varies)
Interval	Varies from 1 to 3 minutes
Duration	Varies greatly; longer with first baby; perhaps from 30 minutes to 2 hours

Please note: All of these figures are approximate.

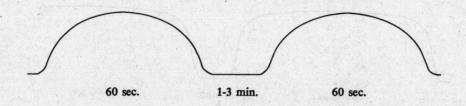

60 sec.   1-3 min.   60 sec.

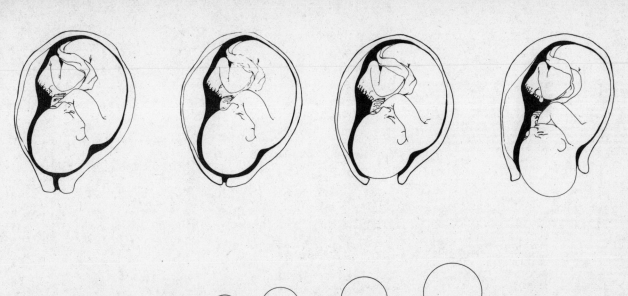

1 2 3 4 5 6 7 8 9 10

Labor and Delivery

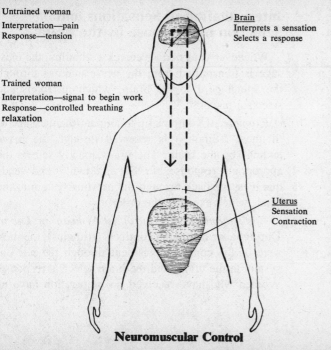

Untrained woman

Interpretation—pain
Response—tension

Trained woman

Interpretation—signal to begin work
Response—controlled breathing relaxation

Brain
Interprets a sensation
Selects a response

Uterus
Sensation
Contraction

Neuromuscular Control

Chapter Four:
Relaxation Techniques

Basic Neurological Principles Applied to Childbirth

This chapter is a discussion of the basic principles of the Lamaze method. The scientific principles are interesting and successful. As far as you are concerned, however, their application to your particular role in childbirth is simple.

1. *Stimulus Response*. The brain receives and interprets a stimulus, then seeks a response to it. During childbirth your brain receives the *stimulus* of the contraction and interprets it either as a pain or a signal to begin your work. It then selects a response of either tensing or relaxing with controlled breathing.

2. *Conditioned response*. Through repeated practice, your relaxation and breathing will become an automatic response to the contractions you experience during childbirth.

3. *Threshold of pain*. You will approach labor with a positive perception of childbirth, which will help to raise your threshold of pain. The intensity of contractions will assume second place to your ability to assume an active and productive role in childbirth.

4. *Distraction*. Because your brain can concentrate effectively on only one sensation at a time, the distraction element of adding more stimulus helps reduce your perception of the intensity of your contractions. Your breathing, relaxation, and the active, supporting role of your husband (massaging, talking, coaching, directing, etc.) help distract your attention from concentrating solely on the sensation of the contraction.

Interpretation of Sensations and Selection of Response by the Brain

Whenever your body receives a stimulus, the message is transmitted from the nerve endings through the spinal cord to the brain, which interprets and selects a response.

Example: If you pick up a hot pan, the message of the heat (stimulus) is received through the nerve endings by the brain. The brain quickly selects the appropriate response of ''Set it down!'' and sends this message back through the nervous system to the hand, which executes the order.

Application to an Untrained Woman in Labor. During labor the uterus contracts (stimulus); the message of the contraction is sent through the nervous system to the brain, and the brain selects a response. Women who have received no preparation have no specific response ready, so the brain is forced to select the most basic of responses: tension. Unfortunately, tension increases the sensation of pain.

Application to a Trained Woman in Labor. During labor the message of the contraction (stimulus) is sent to the brain, which has been trained to interpret the contraction as a strong sensation that must be responded to with controlled relaxation and correct breathing.

Conditioned Response

Through constant repetition, the brain can be taught to respond to a stimulus with a specific response.

Example. When you first learn to drive, a red light is a signal for a confusing array of operations. Each movement of braking, clutching, and shifting gears must be thought out individually. When you become experienced (conditioned) in driving, a red light is your signal to perform the functions smoothly and automatically.

Application to an Untrained Woman in Labor. Through the lurid tales of her friends, movies, books, etc., the average woman has come to associate birth with pain. When she begins her own labor, she is conditioned: her brain interprets "Pain." Even medical personnel unwittingly often reinforce this conditioning. The doctor comes in and asks the mother how her "pains" are. The nurse sits beside her and times the "pains."

Application to a Trained Woman in Labor. The trained woman has repeatedly practiced her relaxation, breathing, and effleurage techniques. When the actual birth takes place, she has conditioned herself to respond automatically to her contractions with these techniques. Her brain has been conditioned to interpret a labor contraction as a strong sensation that opens the cervix, rather than as a pain.

Threshold of Pain

Your brain most effectively registers painful sensations when it is receiving signals from only one strong stimulus at a time. Signals from several strong stimuli act as distracting elements that alleviate or eliminate the sensation of pain. This phenomenon creates a high threshold of pain.

Example. The familiar story of a badly wounded soldier performing feats of courage and strength shows that even a strong sensation of pain can be eliminated by the drive to accomplish what is more important at that time to the soldier.

Application to an Untrained Woman in Labor. The unprepared woman not only expects pain during childbirth but has no response that would be effective in combating the strong sensations emanating from her uterus. She has nothing to concentrate on, nothing to think about, except the contractions which her brain is interpreting as "pain."

Application to a Trained Woman in Labor. The trained woman is equipped with highly active techniques of breathing, neuromuscular control, and effleurage that distract her attention from the intensity of her contractions. Because the trained woman is occupied with other activities, she does not feel the full sensation of the uterine contractions.

Neuromuscular Control (Relaxation)

"Neuro" refers to the nervous system, and "muscular" refers to the muscles of your body. "Control" refers to the ability to make your body do as you bid. You will not be a slave to your contractions but their master.

Why Is Relaxation Necessary?

Tensing during childbirth is a natural response to

the tensing of the uterus. However, tension not only causes exhaustion, oxygen depletion, and a lower pain threshold, but actually prolongs labor physiologically. The hormone that causes your uterus to contract is oxytocin. Adrenaline, the hormone that accompanies the tension-fear-pain syndrome, actually inhibits the effects of oxytocin and makes your contractions less effective. Controlled relaxation helps to shorten labor, conserve energy, decrease pain, and facilitate communication with your husband and the medical team. So remember, the more you tense up during labor, the longer will be your labor. The more you relax, the shorter will be your labor.

Differences between Passive and Active Relaxation

Relaxation usually brings to mind the picture of passiveness—"floating away on a cloud." But, as any woman who has ever had a baby knows, passive relaxation is insufficient to control the intensity of labor contractions. The intensity of the birth experience is of a degree that precludes any possibility of passivity. Birth is active, and must be met by active responses.

How can you differentiate between passive and active relaxation? Try this exercise. First, slowly and with concentration, contract the muscle of your right arm (like Mr. America). Now, let it flop down in a state of limpness. This is passive relaxation. Now, to demonstrate active relaxation, contract the muscle of your arm again, slowly and with concentration, but this time, when you let it down, slowly release, or relax, the muscle with as great a concentration as when you contracted it. Feel your fingers, hand, and arm: are they in a state of relaxation?

Now, imagine that the muscles of your uterus are contracting with greater and greater intensity. Check your arm: is it relaxed? As you imagine the uterine contraction mounting, concentrate on relaxing the muscles of your left arm and then your right and left legs. Check your body: is it relaxed? This is the state of controlled relaxation you want to attain during the intense uterine contractions of labor and delivery.

Muscular Control

During a contraction, the "normal" reaction is to tense your body. As your uterus contracts, the rest of your body, from your feet to your face, tenses right along with it. The uterus, in a sensitive state, is irritable to anything working against it. The normal response of tensing contributes to the traditional pain associated with childbirth.

Since the contractions of the uterus are beyond your power to control, you will have to learn to control the other muscles of your body. You will have to work especially hard during labor to keep the muscles of the pelvic floor in a state of controlled relaxation. During delivery, the baby must pass through the vaginal opening in the pelvic floor. If the muscles surrounding the vagina are tensed, the exit is painful. If these muscles are relaxed, the exit is much easier. You must consciously relax the abdominal muscles during labor. During delivery, however, these are the muscles you are going to use in your bearing-down efforts to expel the baby. As the normal response during contractions is to tense your whole body, you must learn to control not only the muscles of your pelvic floor and the abdomen but also the rest of your body.

To control the various muscles of your body, you must first learn to identify and differentiate them. Lie on your back with a couple of pillows under your head and under your knees. Contract your whole body, one part at a time, and, in the same sequence, relax each part. Begin with your feet. Contract your feet (but don't point them; you might get a cramp), calves, thighs, buttocks, hands, arms, shoulders, neck, and face. Now, as consciously as you tensed them, relax each muscle in sequence. Relax your feet, calves, thighs, buttocks, hands, arms, shoulders, neck, and face. Do this several times until you get the "feel" of your muscles, both contracted and relaxed. Remember, each time you tense or relax a muscle it must be done consciously, not mechanically. Concentrate on your relaxation as one of the techniques that will aid you during delivery.

You have now learned to differentiate the muscles of your body and to contract and relax them with control. To go one step further, you will learn to contract one muscle while relaxing all other muscles. In the same position as before, contract one arm and, as consciously as you tensed that arm, make the rest of your limbs relax. If possible, have your husband give you these directions: "Contract your right arm; relax your left arm and legs." Practice this same exercise, contracting the left arm and relaxing the other limbs. Contract the left leg. Remember that

you are concentrating on relaxing the other limbs; do not concentrate on the contracting one. In labor it will be your uterus that is contracting automatically, and you will have to work hard to make the rest of your body relax.

The next step is to learn to contract two limbs and relax two others at the same time. Contract your right arm and right leg; now, as consciously as you contracted them, relax the left arm and the left leg. Now reverse. After that, try contracting both legs and relaxing both arms. Finally, contract both arms while relaxing both legs.

The last series of muscular control exercises is to contract and relax opposites. Contract your right leg and left arm, then consciously relax your left leg and right arm. You will probably find this set harder than the others, but with practice you will master it. Now reverse, and contract your left leg and your right arm while relaxing the opposites.

No, you are not going to be lying in the labor

room flexing your left leg, etc., to impress the nurse with your flexibility. These exercises merely teach you to relax certain sets of muscles while other muscles are contracting so that in labor, when your uterus is contracting, you will be able to relax the other muscles of your body at will.

Muscular Control During Delivery

During delivery you are interested in keeping the muscles of the pelvic floor (uretha, vagina, and rectum) relaxed. Unfortunately, these are just the muscles that are most likely to tense and that need your greatest control. Remember, your constant practice now will condition you for your baby's birth.

Contraction Simulation

Although we cannot begin to tell you what a contraction feels like, we can provide an exercise that will give you an idea of what it is like to feel a simulated force outside your body, of which you have no control, while allowing you to remain in control of the rest of your body. While you are practicing a contraction, have your husband or partner place his hands above your knee (or on the inside of your thigh) and slowly exert pressure, building it up slowly, simulating a contraction. Although you cannot control this outside force, concentrate on relaxing the rest of your body. You can control the rest of your body (your right arm, your left arm, your right leg, your left leg, etc.).

Neuromuscular Control Exercises

Practice these exercises twice daily, once in the morning and once in the evening. If possible, practice with your partner during the evening session so that you become conditioned to his directions. He can check your relaxation. In this way you become conditioned to his coaching.

As you practice, remember that the muscles you are contracting (be they in arms or legs) are simulating the contractions of the uterus during labor, and the muscles you are relaxing are simulating the rest of your body that you are working to keep relaxed during a contraction. While practicing, concentrate on the relaxed muscles. Relaxation (not tensing) will be your goal during labor.

1. Contract each muscle (feet, calves, thighs, buttocks, pelvic floor, hands, arms, shoulders, and face) in sequence. Relax each muscle in sequence.

2. Contract one muscle; relax three others:
   Contract right arm; relax left arm and both
   legs.

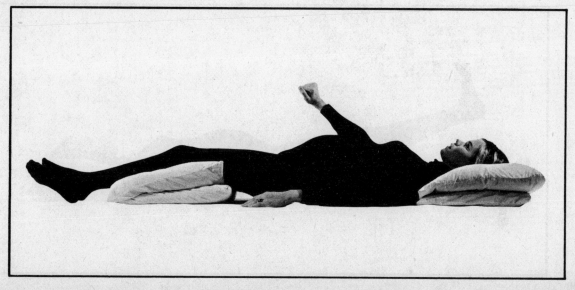

Contract right leg; relax left leg and both arms.

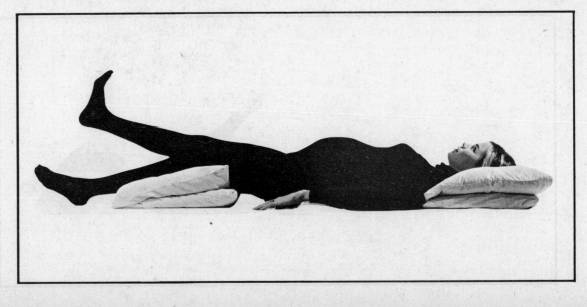

Contract left arm; relax right arm and both legs.

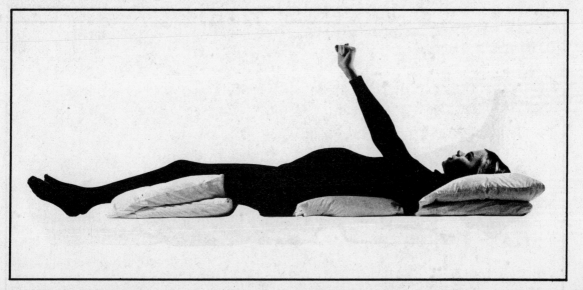

Contract left leg; relax right leg and both arms.

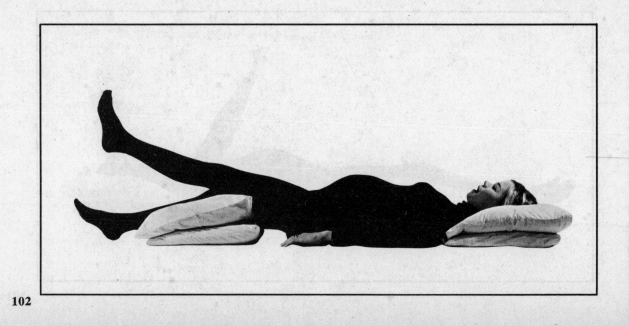

3. Contract two muscles; relax two:
   Contract right leg and right arm; relax left leg
   and left arm.

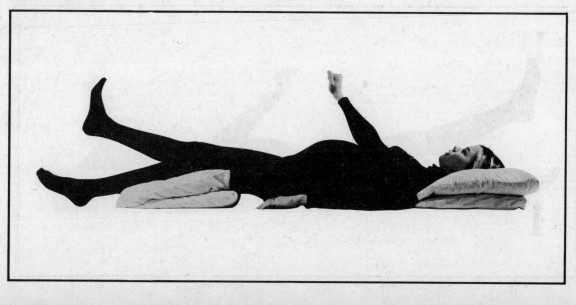

Contract left arm and left leg; relax right arm
and right leg.

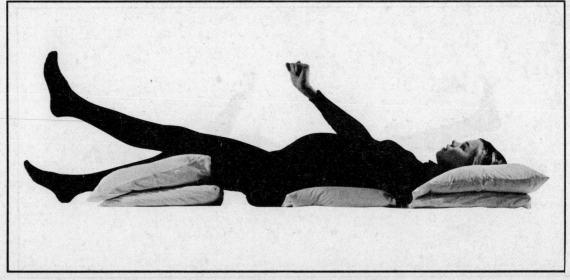

Contract right and left arms; relax right and left legs.

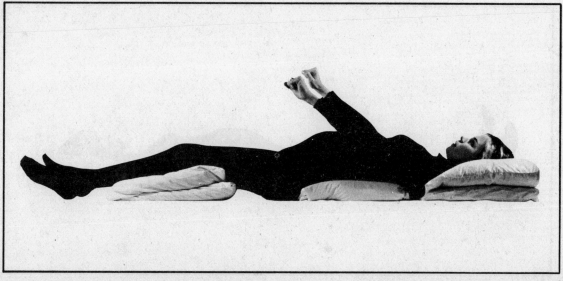

Contract right and left legs; relax right and left
arms.

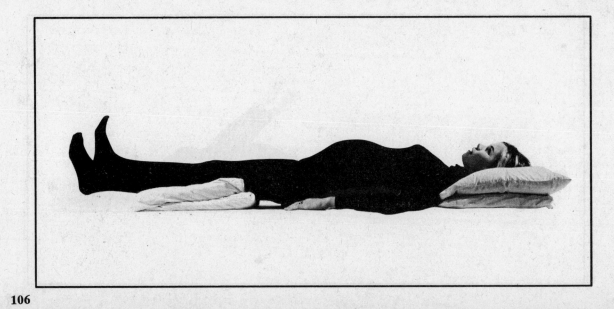

4. Contract opposites; relax opposites:

Contract right arm and left leg; relax left arm and right leg.

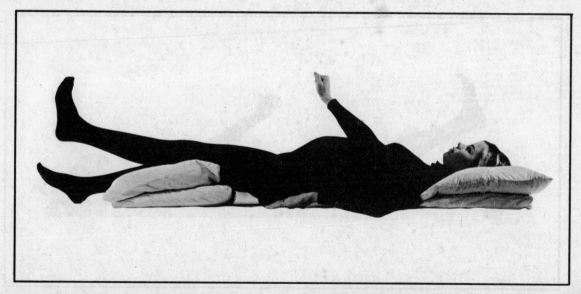

Contract left arm and right leg; relax right arm and left leg.

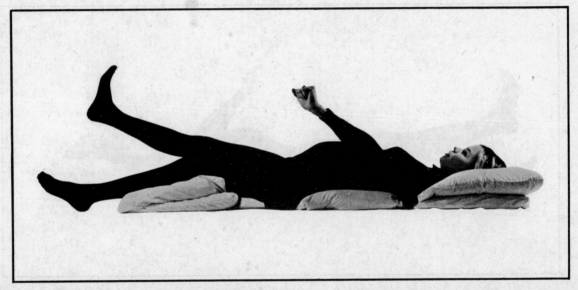

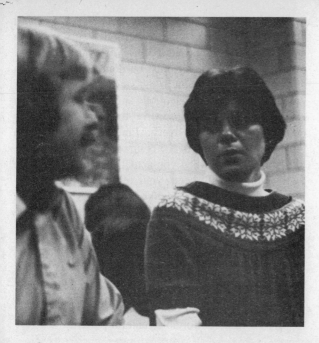

Chapter Five: Breathing Techniques

At the beginning of the book we said that the Lamaze method of prepared childbirth is based upon three main principles:

1. You learn what is going to happen to your body during labor and delivery.

2. You learn techniques that help you remain in control.

3. You practice these techniques so that when you go into labor and delivery you will automatically perform properly and effectively.

Controlled Respiration

You have learned that when you go into labor the contractions of your uterus are going to efface and dilate your cervix. This can be accomplished only by strong, powerful contractions. An untrained woman has never been taught how to respond. But, of course, as with any stimulus of this intensity, she must respond. The natural thing for her to do is to tense up, hold her breath, and clench her teeth. Each of these things works in conflict with the contractions to cause discomfort.

Therefore, it is necessary that you learn a correct response to the contractions you will experience during labor and delivery. You are going to learn to respond to your contractions with a very conscious, controlled type of breathing that will do two things for you. First, controlled breathing will give you something to do during a contraction that is an active response balanced with the increasingly active contractions. Instead of concentrating on the uterine contractions, you will concentrate on your breathing and relaxation. Second, it will keep a balanced amount of oxygen and carbon dioxide in your system.

Just as you were taught to keep an active and conscious control of your relaxation, you want to be in active and conscious control of your breathing. All of your practicing must be done with conscious effort in direct relation to the stages of labor. Never practice without conscientious application. Condition yourself to respond properly to your contractions during labor and delivery. Practice every day in meaningful relation to the contractions you will have in labor, so that when you actually go into labor you will automatically begin your relaxation and breathing techniques with each contraction. To you, a contraction will be a signal to begin your breathing and controlled relaxation.

Key Words

The key words for controlled respiration are:
Slow—in a comfortable, natural pattern;

Even—to ensure an adequate balance of oxygen and carbon dioxide;

Rhythmic—to help with concentration;

Individualized—to meet your needs;

Comfortable—not labored or exhausting; and

Relaxed—each exhalation means conscious relaxation.

There is no one right way. Every woman has her own pattern that works for her.

Breathing Function

To properly understand your breathing function, look at the chart. Breathe in (inhale) to get air into the lungs and breathe out (exhale) to get air out of the lungs. Look closely at the chart. When you breathe in, your chest swells with the filled lungs; when you breathe out, your chest sinks.

Between the lungs and the contents of the abdomen is a thin, flat, disclike muscle called the diaphragm. As you breathe out, it comes up. When you are in labor you are interested in keeping the pressure of this diaphragm off the uterus. You do this by keeping your lungs only partially filled with air—by light chest breathing. When you are in delivery, you will keep your lungs as full as possible, using the pressure of the diaphragm as an aid in expelling the baby.

Put your hands under your breasts, between your abdomen and lungs and pretend that your hands are your diaphragm. Breathe in and your hands go down with the pressure of the filled lungs. Breathe out and your hands come up with the deflated chest.

Try this several times so that you understand the movement of the diaphragm.

Hints on Breathing

1. Do not start your controlled breathing until absolutely necessary. (Conserve energy)

RESPIRATION

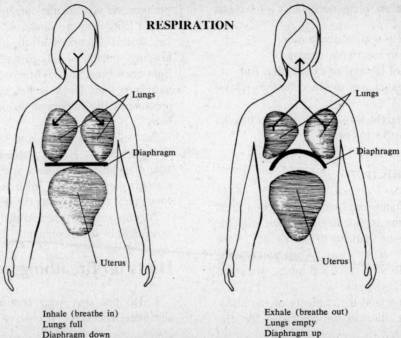

Inhale (breathe in)
Lungs full
Diaphragm down

Exhale (breathe out)
Lungs empty
Diaphragm up

112

2. Stay with first stage breathing as long as possible. Do not proceed to the next stage until you need it. (Gives you the feeling that you still have tools in reserve.)

3. First stage breathing is your basic breathing pattern. If you go through labor using only this first stage, good!

4. Always return to the first stage whenever possible, or when other breathing patterns do not work.

5. Always work hand-in-hand with the intensity of your contractions and the intensity of your breathing response.

6. Always try to keep your breathing as slow and quiet as possible.

7. Because a woman in labor tends to breathe too fast, too hard, and too loud, her coach should be prepared to constantly slow down, calm down, and quiet her breathing.

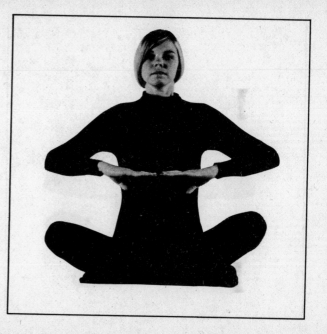

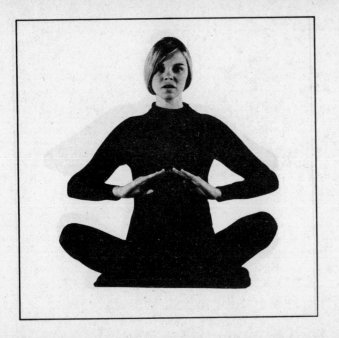

Focal Point

Another technique you can use to increase your stock of tools is the *focal point*. Because the brain can efficiently process only one stimulus at a time, concentrating on a focal point helps to increase your threshold of pain and decrease your perception of the contraction.

Before beginning your breathing exercises, choose an object that is interesting and colorful. Place it at a comfortable distance. As each contraction begins, focus on the point and use it to center all your concentration.

First Stage Breathing

Your first breathing response to your contractions will be a comfortable, relaxed, deep chest breathing.

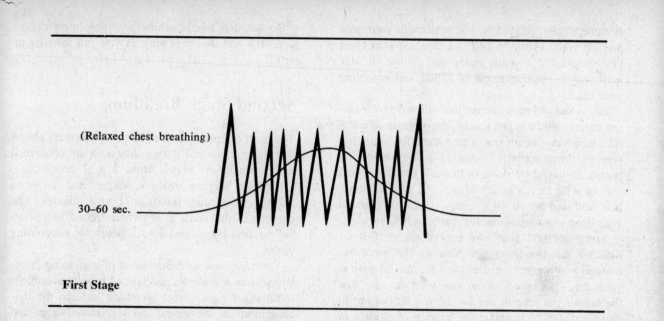

(Relaxed chest breathing)

30–60 sec.

First Stage

Breathe a deep, relaxed breath, in through your nose and out your mouth. As you look down at your chest you should see it gently rising and falling. It may help you to think in terms of filling and emptying your bra.

Begin and end each contraction with a deep cleansing breath, which is just a slow, deep breath in and a full, emptying breath out. The pattern for your first type of breathing will consist of a deep cleansing breath, followed by slow, deep chest breathing, and ending with the cleansing breath. As your contraction will last up to 60 seconds, you will practice your deep chest breathing for that length of time.

You must find your own rate of speed. But remember that the faster you breathe, the more exhausted you become. A slow, steady, natural pace is your aim—not speed. Also, you must be sure that the breath you take in and the air you let out are in equal amounts to maintain the balance of oxygen in your system.

Do not start this breathing until absolutely necessary. Try and use it as long as you can throughout birth.

Second Stage Breathing

The chart of contractions of labor and delivery shows that the contractions during dilatation are concerned with opening the cervix from 3 to 7 centimetres. They have become stronger, longer, and harder to manage. They may last from 1 to 3 minutes. The duration of this phase is anywhere from 5 to 9 hours for the first baby, and 2 to 5 hours for succeeding births.

Your response to contractions of increasing intensity will be a shallow, accelerated type of breathing: *shallow* (or light chest) breathing to keep the diaphragm up off the uterus, and *accelerated* (a gradual build-up in speed) to match the mounting intensity of

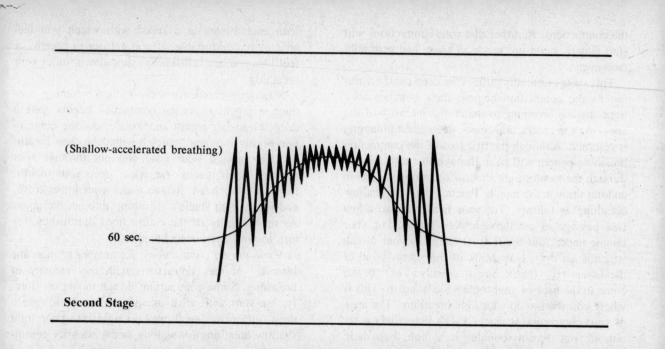

(Shallow-accelerated breathing)

60 sec.

Second Stage

the contractions. Remeber that your contractions will start slowly, build up, reach an apex, and gradually fade away.

This stage essentially utilizes the deep chest breathing as the contraction begins, then switches to a light shallow breathing to match the intensity of the apex. As the contractions ease, deep chest breathing is resumed. Although the first part of the contraction breathing pattern will be in through the nose and out through the mouth, light shallow breathing is done in and out through the mouth. Practice the light shallow breathing as follows: Tilt your head back to allow free passage of air through your throat. Put your tongue under your upper front teeth (so your mouth will not get dry). Now think of the silent sound of the letter ''H'' (huh). Say it silently. Feel the air come in the back of your throat. Say it again. This is where you want to do your light breathing. The apex of your contraction is reached with light shallow in, out, in, out, breath sounding huh, huh, huh, huh,

with each breath at a speed with which you feel absolutely comfortable. If you get out of breath, or feel like you are suffocating, slow down; quiet your breathing.

Now let's practice a second stage breathing contraction together. As the contraction begins, take a deep, cleansing breath and exhale. As the contraction begins to mount, match it with deep chest breathing (in through your nose and out through your mouth). As it reaches the apex, open your mouth, tilt back your head, tongue under your upper teeth, and begin light shallow breathing through the apex. As the intensity of the contractions diminishes, return to your deep chest breathing.

Variation on contractions: Remember to meet the intensity of the contractions with the intensity of breathing. Some contractions do not mount up slowly, but start with great intensity. You would take a deep, cleansing breath and go right into your light shallow breathing for as long as the intensity continues. Some contractions begin slowly, reach an apex, let off, and without warning, hit another peak. You would meet this contraction with a deep, cleansing breath, deep chest breathing, light shallow breathing. Remember, work hand-in-hand with your contractions. Light shallow breathing is not panting, but a controlled, slowly accelerated light breathing. Speed is not your goal, because breathing too fast may cause exhaustion and hyperventilation (an imbalance of oxygen and carbon dioxide in your system). Concentrate on keeping your breathing slow, controlled, relaxed, rhythmical, and quiet.

Third Stage (Transition) Breathing

Look at the chart on page 85 again. The purpose of the contractions during transition is to finish opening the cervix and to begin the expelling phase. These contractions are extremely strong and difficult to manage. They may last anywhere from 60 to 90 seconds and have shorter intervals between them. Although this phase usually lasts only a short time, it is quite intense and exhausting.

Transition breathing is like the second stage shallow light breathing, but with forced blowing out at intervals.

The blowing out is useful in two ways. First, it empties your lungs and pulls up your diaphragm; your back is pressed against the bed and your pubic area is pulled up, tending to shorten the pull over the abdomen and relieve the pressure from the uterus. Second, during the transition contractions you may experience a surprising desire to push the baby out or you may feel that you need to have a bowel movement. This means that your baby has descended and is pressing against your rectum. As your cervix is not completely dilated, it is undesirable for you to push, so to keep from pushing you blow.

To practice a transition contraction, begin with a

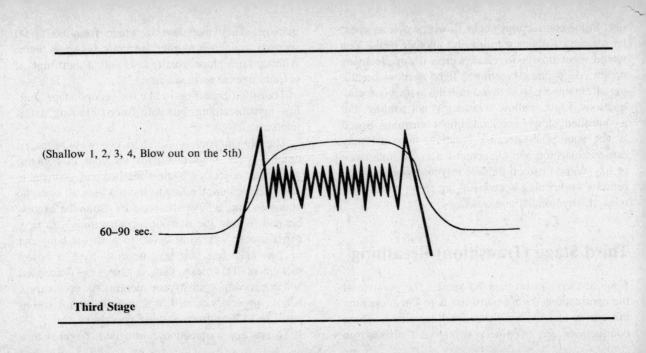

(Shallow 1, 2, 3, 4, Blow out on the 5th)

60–90 sec.

Third Stage

cleansing breath. Take four light shallow breaths, counting as you exhale (breathe in, count 1 as you breathe out; breathe in, count 2 as you breathe out; breathe in, count 3 as you breathe out; breathe in, count 4 as you breathe out). Now breathe in another shallow breath, and as you exhale blow out forcefully through your mouth, as if you were blowing to cool a spoonful of hot soup. Return to your four light breaths, counting 1, 2, 3, and 4 as you exhale, then another light breath and blow out forcefully. Keep up this pattern as long as the contraction lasts, and finish with another deep cleansing breath.

Remember as you practice that these contractions are the most difficult to control. The transition is hard for almost every woman, no matter how many babies she may have had. The saving factors are that this stage usually lasts only a short time and it is an indication that soon you will be giving birth to your baby.

This is the most difficult stage to control, and you will need a great deal of determination, plus moral support and physical assistance from your partner.

Expulsion (Delivery) Breathing

After the transition, your baby is ready to be born. The cervix is opened and the baby's head is far down into the birth canal; now you must push to expel your baby. The contractions continue, but their intensity has decreased. The "muddled" sensation of the transition phase is gone. Although you may have become exhausted during the transition, now you probably will feel as if you have had a shot of adrenalin. The hardest work of labor is over and you are delighted to have come along so far. At last you will begin your active work. The fact that the birth of the baby is near makes this the most exciting and fulfilling part of labor.

When you are in the delivery room the doctor will tell you to push. To push most effectively, you fill your lungs with air (diaphragm down), bear down with your abdominal muscles, and, relaxing the pelvic area, push the baby out through the vaginal opening.

Your position for pushing in the delivery room is to grasp the handles on the delivery table, have your husband or the nurse hold and support your shoulders, curve the shoulders, and keep elbows out, head up, and eyes open. You can practice everything *except the actual pushing* at home, either in your usual position (with pillows under your head and legs) or lying flat on the floor with your legs resting on the seat of a chair.

During delivery, your pushing is most effective at the apex of the contraction, when the cervix reaches its maximum opening. To allow your contraction to reach its apex, your doctor will have you take in two slow breaths and then begin to push. As you practice, mentally give yourself the directions: breathe in, breathe out, breathe in, breathe out. Breathe in (diaphragm down); come up from your practice position; grab under your knees, legs wide apart, shoulders rounded, elbows out, chin up, and eyes open; and begin pushing. Bear down with the abdominal muscles, relax the pelvic area, and push down and out the vaginal opening. Hold your breath for as long as possible. When you can no longer hold it, exhale, take another deep breath, and push again.

You will push only during a contraction. Between contractions you will relax and recuperate as much as possible. *Note: strenuous pushing during the latter stages of pregnancy can be harmful. When you practice this exercise, do not push—just practice holding your breath.*

Pushing Position: It is generally agreed that nature intended squatting to be the most effective and comfortable position for a woman delivering a baby. Unfortunately, not many hospitals allow us to deliver in this way. However, think of yourself in the squatting position and try to simulate as much as possible on the delivery bed. Shoulders rounded, back flat on the bed, your pubic bone rocked forward (the pelvic tilt), will give you the most effective pushing position. Remember to ask your doctor or nurse for advice on the most effective position.

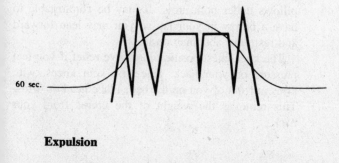

60 sec.

Expulsion

Your first pushes will produce a small patch of hair visible at the opening. With succeeding pushes the baby's head will "crown," that is, the largest part of his head will emerge. As the diameter of the baby's head is a little larger than the vaginal opening there is the possibility that if you push during the crowning you may tear the delicate tissue (called the *perineum*) between the vagina and the rectum. To prevent this, you will stop your pushing at the "crowning," consciously relax the pelvic floor, and let the doctor deliver the head.

To be able to stop pushing in the middle of the contraction with the baby's head about to emerge takes a great deal of practice. Of course, this will be effective only if your doctor agrees ahead of time to give you the verbal order "Stop," for it is only his oral direction that will guide you at that time. To practice this exercise, repeat the pushing for a regular expulsion contraction: breathe in, breathe out, breathe in, breathe out, breathe in, and begin your pushing. In the middle of the contraction, imagine your doctor's order to stop. At this command, stop pushing, release your legs, lie back, open your mouth wide, and begin to pant. This is the only time during labor that you do this type of breathing.

Positions

There are many pushing positions other than the traditional semi-lying one. Choose the one that is most comfortable for you. Research shows that labor in the side-lying position is more comfortable and also more conducive to effective contractions. To tilt the pelvis, place your upper leg in a bent or flexed position perpendicular to your body with several pillows under it for support to maintain good circulation. Roll a pillow and tuck it in against your back so you will have support to lean on. Ask for pillows to place under your uterus or against your chest if this makes you comfortable. Always be ready to change positions, because to do so makes labor more effective.

Another position, sitting upright and supported by pillows allows gravity to help your baby move down. Lean slightly forward with your legs in a comfortable position. Ask for a pillow for back support and pillows under both arms. It may be comfortable to have a pillow in your lap so you may lean forward and rest your abdomen on it.

The knee-chest position may give relief if you feel pressure on your back. Kneel on your knees, with arms in front of you on the bed. Place head on arms. This removes the weight of the uterus from your back.

Breathing Exercises

Whenever you go through the exercises, rehearse in your mind the labor and delivery of your baby. Start with the effacement and continue through dilatation, transition, and delivery. Never practice without relating your controlled breathing and relaxation to the phase and quality of the contraction you are rehearsing. In essence, you are rehearsing your labor and delivery much as an actress rehearses her role. When she enters the stage on opening night, she has been so conditioned to the role that she will perform automatically. And so you must rehearse your role, so that on your "opening night" you too will perform automatically. Each contraction will be your signal for you to begin controlled relaxation and breathing.

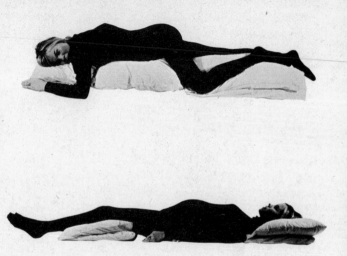

Effacement—Slow, Deep Chest Breathing

Start with a deep cleansing breath, follow with slow, deep chest breathing, and end with a deep cleansing breath. Use six to nine breaths for the duration of the contraction, which is about 60 seconds.

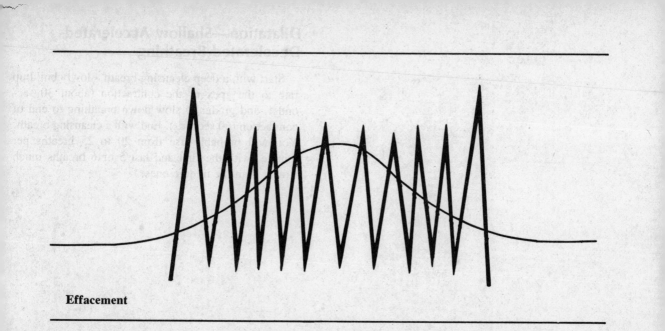

Effacement

Dilatation—Shallow Accelerated-Decelerated Breathing

Start with a deep cleansing breath, slowly build up rate to the apex of the contraction (about 30 seconds), and gradually slow down breathing to end of contraction (60 seconds). End with a cleansing breath. You will probably use from 20 to 25 breaths per minute, with the first and last 5 or 6 breaths much slower than the middle ones.

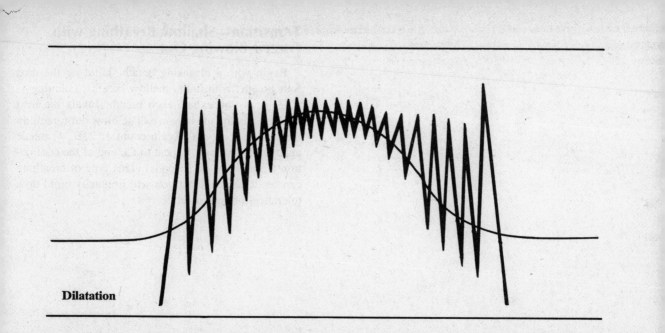

Dilatation

Transition—Shallow Breathing with Forced Blowing Out

Begin with a cleansing breath, build up the next four breaths with light, shallow breaths, counting 1, 2, 3, 4 as you exhale each breath. Inhale the next shallow breath, and as you exhale blow out forcefully through your mouth. Again count 1, 2, 3, 4, inhale again and blow out. Repeat to the end of the contraction (from 30 to 60 seconds). This type of breathing can be exhausting, but you will gradually build up a tolerance through practice.

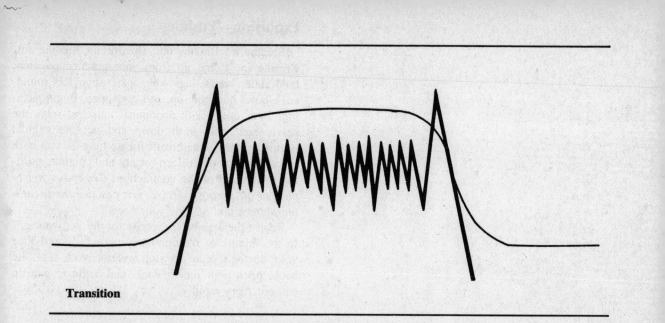

Transition

Expulsion—Pushing

Breathe in. Breathe out. Breathe in. Breathe out. Breathe in. Come up from your practice position; hold under knees, legs wide apart, shoulders rounded, elbows out, chin up, and eyes open. Begin pushing. Bear down with abdominal muscles, relax the pelvic area, and push down and out the vaginal opening. Hold your breath for as long as you can, exhale, take another deep breath, and continue pushing to the end of the contraction. *Remember not to push at all during exercise; just practice the breathing pattern and holding your breath.*

Repeat the expulsion exercise for the "crowning." In the middle of the contraction mentally verbalize your doctor's order to stop, release your legs, lie back, open your mouth wide, and begin to pant in and out, very rapidly.

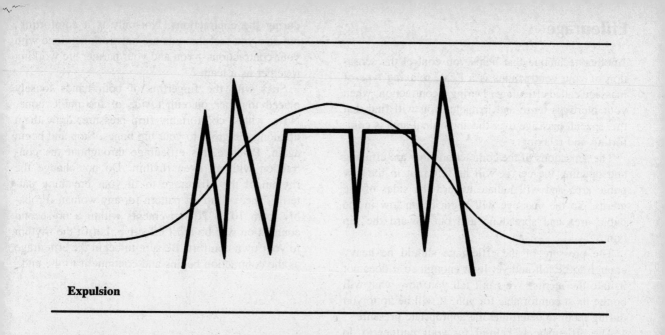

Expulsion

Effleurage

Another technique that helps you control the sensation of your contractions is a light, relaxing type of massage called effleurage. During a contraction, when your uterus is tense and irritable, you will find that this special massage over the abdominal area is comforting and relaxing.

The sensations of the contractions that are effacing and opening the cervix will be felt first in the low pubic area and will radiate toward the sides of the uterus. So the massage will begin down low in the pubic area and spread up and out toward the hip bones.

The pressure of the effleurage should be heavy enough to be felt and yet light enough so it does not irritate the uterus. We can't tell you now what will be the most comfortable for you. It will be up to you during labor to determine the appropriate pressure.

The effleurage is helpful for your partner to do during the contractions. Not only is it comforting, but also you feel that you are not working alone with your contractions—you and your partner are working together as a team.

Start with the fingertips of both hands loosely placed together on either side of the pubic bone. Now, with a comfortably firm pressure, draw them up along the groin to your hip bones. Stop and begin again. Practice this effleurage throughout the contraction with an even rhythm. Do not change the rhythm of the effleurage to fit your breathing patterns. There is no set pattern for any woman. Probably from 10 to 20 movements within a 60-second contraction will be most effective, but fit the rhythm to your own comfort. Be sure to begin the effleurage as the contraction begins and continue it to the end.

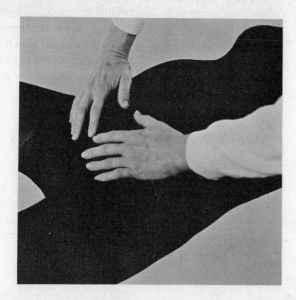 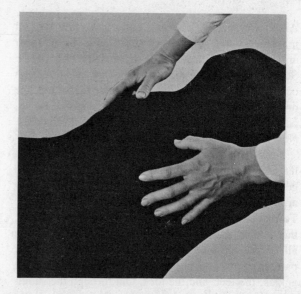

Stroking

Another especially effective and comforting type of massage is the stroking of the thighs, legs, upper arms, and arms—firm, gentle strokes with both hands. Start at the top of the thigh (where most tension occurs). Place one hand on the outer thigh and one on the inner thigh. Firmly and gently stroke down, past the knee over the calf, and out through the toes. Now stroke the other thigh firmly and gently.

Now begin on the upper shoulder, placing both hands on the outer and inner sides of the arm and gently and firmly stroke down through the upper arm, elbow, lower arm, and out through the fingers. To make the stroking most effective and distracting, the woman must consciously concentrate on feeling all of the tension go out with the stroking of her partner's hands: "out through the thigh, the calf, the ankles, the feet, and the toes. Out through the shoulder, the elbow, the wrist, and the fingers."

You will probably spend a good deal of your labor lying on your side. Especially effective is a deep pressure stroking from the coccyx (or tailbone) to the lower back. Place your fingers as far down the tailbone as possible and draw up in a slow, strong, and rhythmic rate. This technique is especially good if you have any discomfort in your back.

Massage

Massage is a rhythmical pressure applied in circular motions. It helps to release muscle tension, increase circulation in the muscles, and provide counterpressure in areas of discomfort. It is important that the woman concentrate on relaxing through the pressure of the massaging hands.

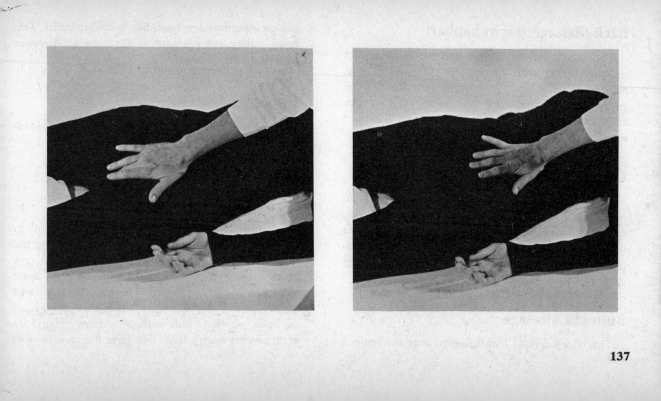

Back Massage (sacro lumbar)

The woman lies on her side and the coach applies pressure (either with the palm of the hand or with hand made into a fist). With circular movements, the coach applies pressure on both sides of the upper spine at the points that give the woman the most relief.

Coccyx Massage (lower spine)

The coach places a hand or fingers over the lowest bones of the spine (called the coccyx) and with slow, strong movements draws both hands up about six inches and then begins again. This movement applies counter pressure against the coccyx and gives great relief.

Buttocks Massage

The coach applies firm massage over the buttock muscles in a manner much like kneading bread. This helps relieve the pressure of the baby as it moves against the rectal area.

Upper Back Massage

The coach firmly rubs the area around the shoulders to help the woman relax and maintain her rhythmic breathing.

Summary

Remember to match the intensity of your breathing with the intensity of contractions. You may find that your contractions do not resemble the storybook contractions that you have seen in illustrations. Some contractions do not become stronger, but start with great intensity. Some contractions begin slowly, reach an apex, subside, and, without warning, piggyback with another contraction. You have the tools to work with the intensity of your contractions. Practice matching your breathing patterns to these variations in contractions.

Practice a contraction beginning. You begin with a deep cleansing breath and consciously relax your body. Your coach begins the effleurage and rapidly checks the relaxation of your hands and feet. The intensity of your contraction mounts and you begin your shallow-accelerated breathing. Your coach continues with the effleurage, reminding you again to relax, telling you of the progress of your contraction, and giving you moral support. Finally, as the contraction fades away, you decelerate your shallow breathing while your coach continues his effleurage. When the contraction is over you take a deep cleansing breath.

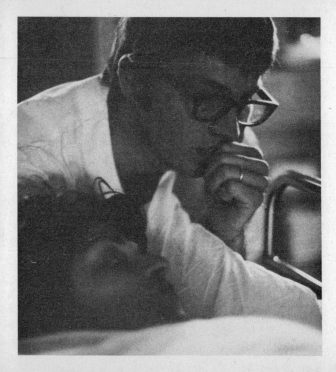

Chapter Six: Father's Chapter

The father? Who needs him? After he's checked his wife in, banish the germ-ridden figure to the waiting room.

This sad picture of the helpless father is fading as men are being prepared to participate and play a vital role in the births of their babies. For years, doctors and nurses have been part of the team that is formed to make sure the mother's delivery is safe, healthy, and happy; now the trained, interested father has joined that team.

Our four Lamaze babies have convinced me that there is a great need for trained fathers. When Donna became pregnant with our first baby in France, we began together to learn about our baby-to-be and how it would enter our lives. We explored concepts of childbearing and slowly gained a good understanding of what lay ahead of us in pregnancy, and

141

what would happen in labor and delivery. We began our Lamaze classes when Donna was seven months pregnant. Almost immediately I was able to help with Donna's breathing and especially her relaxation patterns.

There was something rewardingly different about this way of having babies. The Hollywood image of the father-to-be, uselessly boiling water in the backwoods or ineffectually pacing the echoing corridors of anonymous hospitals, kept recurring to me—in contrast, here I was, aiding my wife and learning how to help her through labor and delivery. By the time our baby was due we were both elated about the prospects. Our instructor had prepared us well, and our doctor had been extremely helpful in making us understand all facets of the imminent delivery. He granted permission for me to both photograph and tape record this exciting first birth.

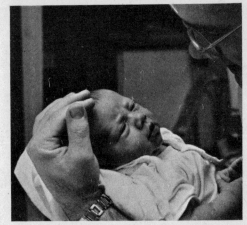

A Lamaze father and infant daughter.

Much of the happiness that shows up in the photographs of Marguerite's birth was there because I was present as husband, friend, and helper. This same joyful atmosphere was present at the births of all our other children.

Though we have excellent hospitals and fine medical staffs, nothing can replace the intimacy and richness of sharing that a trained coach can impart at childbirth. You as a coach can uniquely provide the assistance and support which make up a large part of the Lamaze experience.

Both before and during the birth of your child, knowledge and understanding are the keys to your part in a trained birth. Learn along with the mother what this birth business is about. Attend the Lamaze classes with her. You will be needed to help her learn exercises, breathing, and relaxation. When you attend classes with your wife you *both* learn the Lamaze principles more thoroughly and can profitably ask questions and exchange notes with the instructor and other expecting couples. Your solid understanding will give you both confidence and calm—important elements in a happy delivery.

At the hospital during labor and delivery you will find yourself in the role of husband, protector, monitor, and friend. Many of the things you can do for your wife are *best* done by you—as I see the vital role husbands play in Lamaze-trained childbirths, I wonder more and more how wives ever got along without our assistance.

You will have both physical tasks (effleurage, monitoring your wife's breathing patterns, and checking her relaxation) and psychological tasks (encouraging her, cheering her on, and keeping her informed of her progress). These psychological tasks are fully as vital as your physical work: imagine what effect cheering spectators have on a front-running sprinter or a touchdown-destined quarterback.

So, you say, I have all that to give? Fine, but what do I get out of this? Here is where the human qualities of the Lamaze method come into play. By being a direct, heavily committed participant in the birth of your child, you will gain increased respect and love from your wife.

The birth of a child is one of the most important experiences that can be shared in married life. Your wife needs your help and calls for you. A man who cannot respond to his wife's needs feels helpless and impotent, and his wife cannot help but be disappointed with his inability to respond. By being prepared to help your wife at this time, you will gain tremendous pleasure from your ability to protect and support her. Instead of being condemned to a role of frustrated ignorance and waiting-room impotence, you will gain an honest, lasting feeling of having helped immeasurably in the birth of your child.

The challenge of childbirth provides many men with an opportunity to establish mature, deep relationships with their wives. In this time of stress, a husband's active participation demonstrates that he cares a good deal about what is happening to the woman he loves. He assumes responsibility toward both his wife and the child they have conceived. He shows that he respects his wife's efforts and is willing to share them. He learns to know his wife in one of the most important and creative times in her life. I can say for myself that my joy in being with Donna through all four of our babies' births has extended itself into a rich, busy life of shared activity and mutual respect, one that could not be more fulfilling.

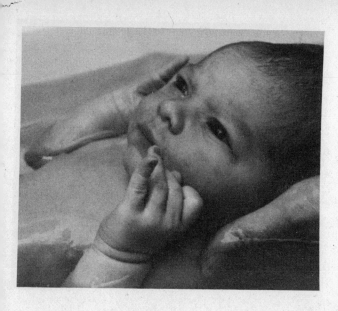

Chapter Seven: The Birth

At last, the big day. For weeks you've been rehearsing. The last week you were beginning to wonder if it ever was really going to happen to you. You've been having many contractions, and at first you thought each time you had one perhaps you were in labor. But each time the contractions went away. You got so that you just ignored them. But this time the contractions are not going away. Little by little you become aware that not only have they stayed but they are becoming increasingly stronger. Perhaps you have a little "bloody show," a small amount of mucous fluid that is released from the neck of the cervix. You might even have a leak in the amniotic sac and feel a small gush of clear fluid. As time passes, you become increasingly aware that "this is it." True labor is identified by regular contractions that become increasingly stronger. Although the contractions of false labor may be regular, they do not increase in intensity.

TRUE (ACTIVE) LABOR CONTRACTIONS (Cervix becomes effaced and dilated)	FALSE (EARLY) LABOR CONTRACTIONS (Cervix uneffaced and closed)
Occur at regular intervals	Occur at regular or irregular intervals
Intervals gradually shorten	Intervals remain long
Intensity gradually increases	Intensity remains same or diminishes
Located mainly in back	Located mainly in abdomen
Intensified by activity	Activity has no effect

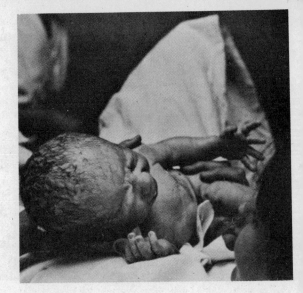

When you are sure you are in labor, call your husband. Like many husbands, he may be more excited and nervous than you are. He will immediately want to call the doctor, the hospital, and the whole world. Let him call the doctor, for the doctor is interested in your contractions and will want to know whether or not there has been any bloody show or leaking water. But don't let your husband talk you into going to the hospital too early in the game. The normal labor lasts 9 hours and the first part takes the longest; it would be nicer to spend it in your own home where you probably have an interesting book to read or a little knitting to finish. Nothing is so boring as a hospital to a person who is not sick. And remember, you are not sick—you are going to have a baby.

If your contractions are light enough for you to take a nap, by all means do so, for rest is important now. You have a big job ahead of you, one that will be the most strenuous task you have ever undertaken. Switch to light liquids such as tea with sugar or honey, soup, or jello that will give you energy.

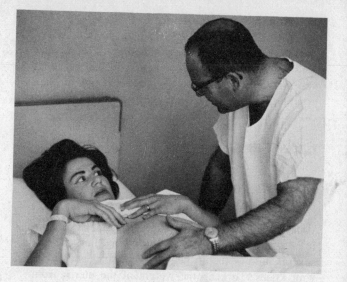

The purpose of these early contractions is effacing, or taking up, the cervix. When the contractions become strong enough that you feel you need to start conscious relaxation and breathing techniques, and you are very sure you are in labor, it is time to pick up your suitcase and head for the hospital.

Early Labor

Mother's Role

You are now taken into the labor room, where your coach is probably waiting for you. Have him roll up the bed so you are not lying flat and get several pillows to put behind your head and under your knees. To keep the weight of the uterus from pressing against your body during labor, assume an almost upright sitting posture or lie on your side. It is healthy to change position from time to time throughout labor. By now you are probably in pretty good labor and will begin to use your relaxation and breathing techniques if you have not already. To be most effective, and least exhausting, the breathing patterns should not be begun until you absolutely need them.

The nurse will come in and examine you. If this is your first baby, the contractions you have been having thus far probably have been working to efface, or thin out, the cervix. Remember, the first stage of labor takes the longest time. Don't become discouraged if you have not progressed as far as you thought. Even though we have tried to describe the sensation of contractions during labor, it is impossible to portray their intensity. Your first contractions may surprise you with their strength.

If you have had other babies, you will probably be dilating by this time. Remember that each contraction is the mechanism by which the cervix is effaced and dilated and your baby is expelled. This early stage is the time to analyze the contractions, so that you become accustomed to their quality, and to condition yourself to respond to each one with your breathing and relaxation techniques. Consciously keep your body, extremities, and pelvic area relaxed.

Continue the first stage deep chest breathing for as long as you can. If you could get all the way through labor with this type of breathing, it would be marvelous, for it is the least exhausting and enervating. Most women begin to use dilatation breathing much too soon in labor.

Coach's Role

Make the mother as calm as possible. Reassure her that she knows what is happening and has techniques to cope with her contractions. Help her with her breathing patterns. Try the effleurage—she will tell you if you are doing it correctly. If effleurage on the uterus is not pleasant, try the deep back massage.

Give her verbal instructions to relax her hands, her feet, and especially her pelvic area. Work with the contractions: learn to recognize the beginning, apex, and end. Ask her to tell you when they begin, when they become harder, and when they let up. As the contractions become very regular, you will learn to recognize these phases on your own. Time the intervals and become familiar enough with them to tell her when a contraction should begin, reach its apex, and end. The effectiveness of the Lamaze technique is due in large part to the distracting elements outside of the contraction, so help the mother to concentrate on her relaxing, breathing, and effleurage. By talking to her you are giving "moral support" and providing an excellent distraction.

Active Labor

The contractions are becoming stronger, longer, and

perhaps harder to manage. They will probably last about 60 seconds, with a rest interval of from 1 to 3 minutes between them. These contractions are working to open the cervix. You begin to feel that controlling the contractions takes more effort. You become extremely busy, and can't be bothered with distractions.

Mother's Role

When the chest breathing is no longer sufficient, switch to the shallow-accelerated breathing. Remember to match your breathing activity to the intensity of the contractions. Keep your breathing slow, regular, and rhythmic and concentrate as much as you can. Consciously control the relaxation of your body, especially the pelvic area. Use the effleurage. You must catch each contraction as it begins and work with it carefully from its beginning, through the apex, to the end. Always keep "on top of" your contractions. Keep them under control. Should you

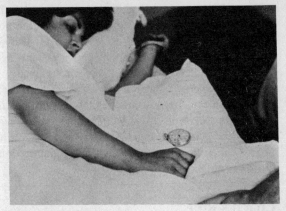

Timing the contractions.

lose control of a contraction, get through it as well as you can. Begin afresh and with renewed concentration on the next one. If at any time you become exhausted in dilatation, or feel that the shallow breathing is no longer sufficient, return to the deep chest breathing for several contractions. When you return to the dilatation breathing, it will be much more effective.

When the membranes rupture, be prepared for a dramatic change in the intensity of your contractions.

Coach's Role

Continue your efforts to keep the mother as comfortable as possible. Time her contractions and direct their progress. Remind her to relax while checking her hands and feet. Use effleurage, unless her uterus is irritable and the effleurage is uncomfortable. Wipe her forehead with a cool cloth and give her small amounts of ice to moisten her throat and lips. Constantly give her direction, encouragement, and moral support. Keep her from breathing too fast. After any examination be sure the nurse or doctor tells her of the progress of her contractions.

Transition

Gradually the quality of your contractions will change. You will find they last longer, are stronger, and have shorter intervals. You will begin to feel an urge to push or perhaps will have a greater difficulty in controlling the contractions and in relaxing.

Mother's Role

If we tell you that you may experience nausea, vomiting, trembling, cramps, backache, or extreme sleepiness at this time, please don't give up. When you have arrived at this phase, it is time to be encouraged, because these are the signs that you have been through it all and the birth of your baby is very close. Although you are not quite dilated completely to 10 centimetres, the expelling forces of your uterus are now coming into play, and the powerful desire to push may feel overwhelming. Because the cervix is not completely opened, you will use transition breathing to help make pushing impossible. As your contraction starts, take a cleansing breath, build up with four shallow breaths, counting 1, 2, 3, 4 as you exhale each breath, inhale another shallow breath, and blow out forcefully. Continue this breathing to the end of the contraction, and end with a cleansing breath. You will have to work particularly hard to relax your body. Effleurage is especially effective. You may find that the side position is the most comfortable for this stage. Remember that, although this is the most difficult stage, it is also usually the shortest. The transition is your signal that you will soon begin your pushing efforts to

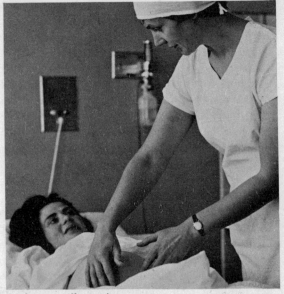

The nurse will examine you.

expel the baby. If you are extremely exhausted at this stage, or if for any reason your transitional stage extends over a long period of time, a local anesthetic may be very welcome. It will help you relax, give you some rest before the strenuous task of delivery, and may speed up your progress.

Coach's Role

Continue what you have been doing. Encouragement is most necessary at this point. Tell the mother how well she is doing. Remind her that each succeeding contraction is getting her closer to the delivery of the baby. Help her to relax between contractions. Be sure she catches each contraction as it starts. Continue using effleurage. Deep back massage is particularly effective during this phase.

It is not uncommon for a woman to begin to lose control during transition. The three key techniques a coach can use to help her regain control are: eye contact, a firm voice, and firm touch. Using a firm voice, speak directly into her ear, place both hands firmly on her face, bring your face down to her, and tell her to open her eyes and look at you. Continue with the command until she does; then tell her to open her mouth, breathe in, and breathe out. You may have to breathe with her. Keep her breathing in and out. Now move your hands to her shoulders and begin to firmly stroke them. Remind her to keep her eyes open and continue her breathing technique. Now begin to stroke the rest of her body. Tell her to relax to the touch of your hands. Give her support, directions, and encouragement.

Expulsion

If this is your first baby, at the end of transition the nurse will probably have you begin pushing in the labor room to get the head of the baby to the exterior opening of the birth canal (the vagina). With your first baby it takes, of course, more pushes to get it through the birth canal and out. You will be delighted to be allowed to push. At last you are doing something that seems to have a real purpose.

Mother's Role

The nurse will probably inform you that with the next contraction you will be allowed to push. As the contraction starts, take a deep breath, let it out; take another deep breath, let it out, take in a deep breath, grasp your legs under the knees, elbows out, chin up, eyes open; bear down with your abdominal muscles out through the vagina. Hold your breath as long as you can, let it out only when you absolutely have to, take in another deep breath, and continue pushing to the end of the contraction. Rest as much as possible during the period between contractions. You will repeat your pushing with each succeeding

contraction until the head of the baby can be seen at the exterior outlet.

If you are to deliver in a delivery room, you will be put on a table and wheeled into the delivery room, where your doctor will be waiting. It is especially difficult to remain in control when you are having contractions on the table, so ask to be allowed to wait if a contraction begins just as you are about to get on or off the table. Do remind yourself that the birth of the baby is so near that extra control is most rewarding. Once in the delivery room you will be transferred to the delivery table. Drapes will be placed over your abdomen and legs. Your pelvic area will be cleansed with warm (we hope) antiseptic solution. Your legs will be placed in stirrups. The nurse will show you where the handles are on the stirrups that you can hold while you push. There is a mirror placed so you can see the birth of your baby. Remind your nurse to adjust it so you can see the baby come out. The nurse will instruct you where to place your body on the delivery table, and all is now ready for the delivery.

The doctor takes his place at the end of the delivery table. The doctor may perform an episiotomy at this time to prevent tearing of the perineal tissue. This consists of a small, painless cut in the anesthetized perineum to allow more room for the baby's head to come through without undue stretching.

As your contraction begins, the doctor will direct you to repeat your pushing as you did in the labor room. If he feels that your pushing is not as effective as it might be, ask him how he thinks you might do better. Remember, the contractions of expulsion are of less intensity than during transition and are much easier to control. Each succeeding push brings you noticeably closer to the birth of your baby.

As you look into the mirror, with each succeeding push you will see more and more of the head at the opening. Finally, when the whole top of his head comes through (the "crowning"), lie back and pant

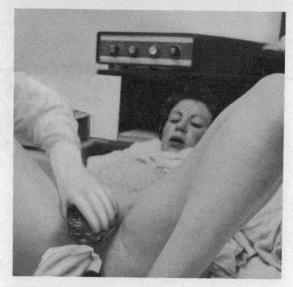

Donna Ewy's delivery.

155

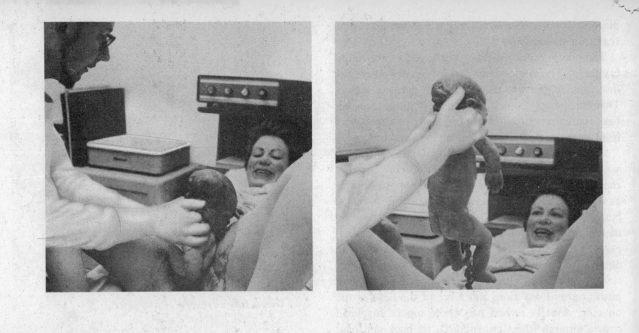

as the doctor delivers the head. You can see your baby's eyes, nose, mouth, and chin, and finally the whole head is delivered. As the head is the most difficult to deliver in the expulsion, your real work is over. The rest of your baby's body comes effortlessly. The doctor will hold your baby down, swab out his nose and mouth, and suction away excess mucus. When he places the baby in your arms, you realize that the long hours of labor were well worth it.

Your work is not quite done, however, for the placenta must be expelled. With the next contraction the placenta, which has detached itself from the walls of the uterus, is expelled. The doctor inspects it to see that no part has remained in the uterus. The nurse begins to massage your uterus to help stop the flow of blood. Your baby is then examined by the doctor, weighed, measured, wrapped in prewarmed clothes, and finally admired by all.

Your work is over. You should be exhausted, but

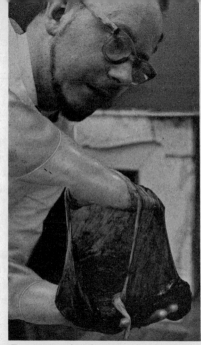

Examining the placenta.

157

both you and your husband are exhilarated by your achievement. The nurse will take you to the recovery room and then to your room in the maternity ward, where you can get a well-earned rest.

Coach's Role

You will give the mother mostly moral support at this time. When the doctor tells her to stop for the crowning of the baby's head, help her to lie back and start her panting. You have worked almost as hard as the mother during labor. Now the "fruits of your labor" are well rewarded by the unique experience of being part of the birth of a child.

Even if you are allowed in the delivery room, you may be asked to leave if any complication (such as a cesarean delivery) should arise. If this should happen, the greatest assistance you can offer will be your cooperation with the medical staff.

Last-Minute Hints

1. Do not start controlled breathing until you absolutely need it. Stay with each stage of breathing as long as you can before you start on the next stage, for each stage is progressively more difficult and tiring.

2. Change your position (lying on your back or side, sitting up, etc.) as often as possible during labor so you don't get bored in one position.

3. Urinate as frequently as you need during the first stage of labor.

4. If you begin to feel that the contractions are coming too fast and hard for you to handle, ask your doctor for some kind of sedation to give you a chance to relax and keep in control. You are not practicing to be a hero.

5. If you find that your dilatation or transitional breathing is becoming ineffective, stop it and resume

the deep chest breathing for several contractions. When you return to the previous breathing pattern, it will be more effective.

6. Bring some type of sour hard candy to give you energy during the arduous task of labor.

7. Bring a snack or packed lunch for your coach—he gets hungry (especially if you have a long labor) and appreciates nourishment.

8. Bring a paper bag with a Chapstick (your lips get quite dry) and talcum powder (for the effleurage). You can also use this paper bag to breathe into should you get hyperventilated.

9. Bring a pair of your husband's warm woolen socks in case your feet get cold during labor.

Suggested Check List for the Hospital Stay

Suitcase:

Nightgowns—if you are breastfeeding, try to get nightgowns that button down the front. You might want to wear the hospital gown the first half day or so.

Bathrobe and slippers.

Bras—(two or three) even if you are not nursing the baby.

Hair care equipment—you probably will want to wash your hair in the hospital if your doctor approves.

Toilet articles—toothbrush and paste, deodorant, cologne, etc.

Change for newspapers, etc.

Baby book—footprints can be put in the book in the delivery room or by the nursery staff.

Camera and film—check with the hospital as to the possibility of taking pictures in the delivery room.

Baby announcements and writing material.

Most pads and sanitary belts are supplied by the hospital.

Tape recorder—if you want to record labor and/or birth.

Evaluation report.

List of important numbers to call with the good news.

Goodie Bag: (Keep this handy in the labor room—use it for hyperventilation.) Something to keep your mouth from becoming too dry—either mouthwash, breath spray, sour candy, lemon or orange slices, or gum.

Lubricant for mouth and nose such as Vaseline or lanolin.

Powder or lotion for back rub or effleurage.

Small baggies—two or three to make ice packs or heat packs in case of back labor.

Pair of extra socks.

Lamaze book

Watch with second hand.

Pack lunch for husband's nourishment.

Homecoming Day:

Have the things you want to wear home as well as the baby's clothes in a place where your husband can easily find them. Be sure and tell him where they are so the night before you are scheduled for dismissal, he can bring them in. This will save wear and tear on both of you.

Dress—something loose and comfortable.

Underwear.

Baby outfit:

   undershirt

   diaper (usually provided by hospital as most use disposables)

   kimono or one-piece stretch outfit

   booties

   cap

   receiving blanket

   outer blanket

Summary—Early Phase (Effacement)

Characteristics

Purpose. To thin out and take up the cervix. Dilatation of cervix to 3 centimetres.

Contractions.

Intensity—light.

Length—30 to 60 seconds.

Intervals—5 to 20 minutes.

Duration—5 to 8 hours with first labor; shorter with second.

Emotional Feelings. Excited and confident.

Physical Signs.

Recurring (increasingly stronger) contractions.

Bloody show (small amount of mucous fluid streaked with blood).

Rupture or leak of the amniotic sac.

Increased urination.

Increased vaginal discharge.

Feeling of menstrual cramps.

"Flu-like" feeling.

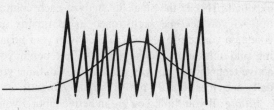

Mother's Role

Breathing. Deep, relaxed chest breathing (start as distraction technique only when absolutely necessary).

Relaxation. Consciously keep body, extremities, and pelvic area relaxed.

Effleurage. Try it.

Position. Keep up your regular activities, but stop

to do your breathing and relaxation when you need it.

NOTE: Remember, each contraction is the mechanism by which the cervix is opened and the baby expelled. This is the stage to analyze each contraction so you become accustomed to its quality and condition yourself to respond to each with your breathing and relaxation techniques. Do not begin your active techniques until you need them. Continue your daily activities, but try not to fatigue yourself.

Eating. If you think you are in active labor, switch from solid foods to nutritious and energy-giving liquids such as orange juice, jello (hot or cold), tea with sugar or honey.

Call your doctor. Try to stay at home during this phase.

Coach's Role

Make the woman as calm as possible:

1. Help determine whether this is early or active labor.
2. Time contractions. Help to ascertain increasing strength.
3. Help the woman rest and get energy for the coming work.

Reassure her that she has learned to cope with her contractions.

Help obtain and adjust pillows.

Help with breathing pattern.

Try effleurage.

Give her verbal directions to relax different areas—especially extremities and pelvic area.

Work with contractions. Learn to recognize beginning, apex, and end. Time intervals and become familiar enough to tell your wife of their progression.

Summary—Active Phase (Dilatation)

Characteristics

Purpose. To open the cervix (3 to 7 centimetres).
Contractions.

Intensity—strong and long, harder to manage, and closer together.

Length—60 seconds.

Intervals—1 to 3 minutes.

Duration—first baby, 5 to 9 hours; other children, 2 to 5 hours.

Emotional Feelings. Contractions take more effort; extremely busy—can't be bothered with extraneous distractions. Toward the end of this stage, may begin to doubt ability to cope and continue throughout birth.

Physical Signs.

More pressure in the pelvic area.

Possible cramps in legs and hips.

May experience a backache.

More difficulty in relaxing.

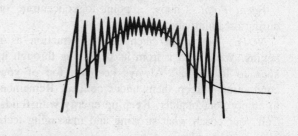

Mother's Role

Breathing: Cleansing breath, then light shallow breathing, end with cleansing breath. Remember to match breathing activities to intensity of contraction. Do not overbreathe.

Relaxation. Consciously keep body relaxed, especially the pelvic area and extremities.

163

Effleurage. Especially effective.

Position. Side and sitting positions with head and back propped up, pillows under legs. Remember to change positions frequently.

Focal Point. Choose a point to concentrate on during breathing and relaxation.

NOTE: You must catch each contraction as it begins. Work with it from its beginning through its apex to its ending. Always keep on top of your contractions—keep them under control. Remember to empty your bladder. Keep up energy with fluids. Tell your coach what stroking and massaging techniques feel good.

Coach's Role

Be sure the woman is in a comfortable position; get pillows if needed.

Time her contractions. Tell her when the contraction should be starting, when it should reach the apex, and when it should end.

Remind her to relax.

Use effleurage, stroking, and massage on pressure points.

Wipe her forehead with a cool cloth if necessary.

Give her small amounts of ice to moisten her throat and lips.

Constantly give her encouragement and moral support.

After each examination, have the nurse tell her of her progress.

Put heat in areas where she feels pressure (i.e., back, thighs, pelvis).

Try cold cloths in pressure areas.

Be sure you are also in a comfortable position.

Keep up your energy with food.

Be sure you get enough liquids.

Be sure to empty your bladder.

Summary—Transition

Characteristics

Purpose. Finish opening cervix (7 to 10 centimetres). Expelling forces come into play.

Contractions.

Intensity—extremely strong and erratic; difficult to manage.

Length—60 to 90 seconds.

Intervals—1 minute (erratic).

Duration—short (anywhere from 5 minutes to 2 hours—40 minutes is average).

Emotional Feelings. Confusion—quality of contractions has changed. Disorientation. Urge to push (or muddled feeling) appears. Discouragement. Difficulty remaining in control.

Physical Signs.

Nausea.

Trembling and perspiration.

Shaking and shivering.

Rectal pressure.

Pressure on pelvic floor.

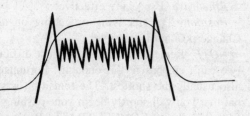

Mother's Role

Breathing. Forced exhalation. Start with cleansing breath, build up light, rapid breathing, then blow out with forced exhalation (as if you were cooling soup on a spoon). Continue with four light breaths, take another shallow breath and blow out to the end

165

of the contraction, and finish with deep, cleansing breath.

Relaxation. Extremely difficult, but important. You will need the utmost help from your coach. Remember that tensing will prolong your labor.

Effleurage. Especially effective.

Position. Try side-lying or getting on all fours. Change position if possible.

NOTE: Remember this is the most difficult stage (we can't emphasize this enough). Fortunately, it is also usually the shortest. The transition is your signal that you will shortly begin your pushing to bring forth your baby. CONCENTRATE! Because of lack of oxygenation this phase will require your most diligent control. It will take special effort, but listen to your coach. Remember, it is to your benefit to respond to directions. Concentrate on getting through one contraction at a time.

Coach's Role

Time contractions and direct their progress: beginning, apex, and end.

Direct the mother to relax.

Use effleurage.

Encouragement and the utmost moral support are most necessary at this time.

Continue to make her as comfortable as possible.

Help her to relax between contractions.

Be sure she catches each contraction as it starts.

Be firm and simple in your directions.

Maintain eye to eye contact.

Don't let intensity frighten you; it is normal.

Summary—Expulsion

Characteristics

Purpose. Expel the baby.
Contractions.
Intensity—return to dilatation strength.
Length—approximately 60 seconds.
Intervals—1 to 3 minutes.
Duration—varies, 30 minutes to 2 hours; sometimes longer with first baby.
Emotional Feelings. Exhilaration—this is the active phase (pushing). Thrill of seeing your own baby born. Sometimes, fatigue.
Physical Signs.
Pressure points change.
Pushing usually gives relief.
May feel baby's movement down birth canal.
May feel rectal pressure and backache.

Some women feel stretching or burning sensation in perineum.

Mother's Role

Breathing. When your doctor tells you to push, breathe in, breathe out, breathe in, breathe out, breathe in, and bear down with your abdominal muscles. Push out the vagina. Take a breath when you need it, again fill your lungs with air, and bear down until the contraction is over.

When the baby's head crowns, push until your doctor tells you to "stop." Lie back quickly and start panting.

Relaxation. Try to keep as relaxed as possible, especially your feet, legs, and pelvic area.

Position. Side-lying or semi-sitting, shoulders rounded, chin off your chest, elbows up and eyes open. Be sure you can see in the mirror. If you can't, the nurse will be glad to adjust it for you.

NOTE: Push with even and controlled pushes at apex of each contraction. Keep face and mouth relaxed. Rest between contractions.

Coach's Role

Bring pillows to delivery room.

Remind the mother to relax.

Show her the abdominal muscles she will use during the pushing.

Hold up her shoulders while she is pushing.

Count with slow, firm voice.

Help her to relax and recuperate as much as possible between contractions.

Be sure she can see in the mirror.

Remind her to keep her chin off her chest and her elbows up.

When the doctor tells her to "stop," help her to fall back and start panting.

Be sure that if the mother desires she receives the baby in her arms for skin-to-skin contact and that if she wishes to breastfeed, the baby is allowed to nuzzle at her breast. Ensure that all of you have special time to get to know each other.

A Lamaze Birth

Five hours after the onset of labor, Ann is admitted to the hospital and the baby's heartbeat is checked. Examination shows that effacement is complete and Ann's cervix is dilated to about two centimetres.

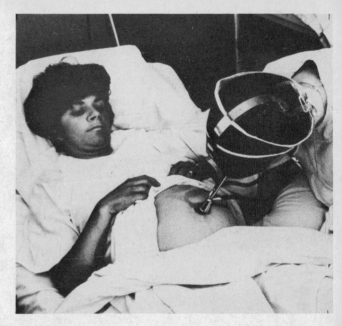

Early dilatation. As each contraction starts, Ann begins her deep chest breathing. Milt uses effleurage and checks her hands and feet for relaxation.

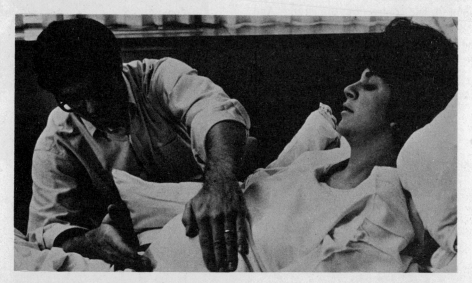

Five centimetres of dilatation. Ann's membranes have been ruptured, and contractions are strong. Ann uses shallow-accelerated breathing; Milt checks her relaxation and gives her deep back massage.

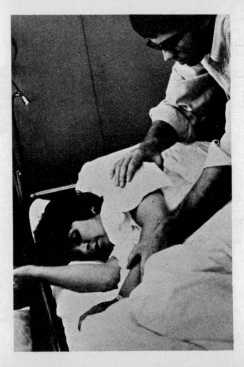

3:45—

Transition. Feeling tremendous pressure on the pelvic floor, Ann uses transitional breathing to counteract her desire to push. Milt, dressed for the delivery room, gives Ann great physical and emotional support.

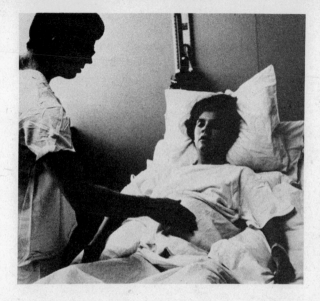

4:15—

The doctor has just examined Ann and found that her cervix is completely dilated. To everyone's delight, she is ready to go to the delivery room.

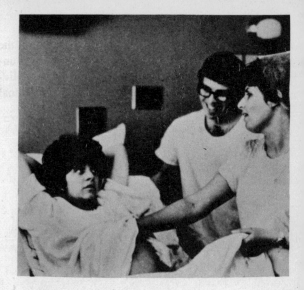

4:40—

In the delivery room the doctor directs Ann to Push! Milt supports Ann's shoulders and cheers her on. With each push, more and more of the baby's head can be seen.

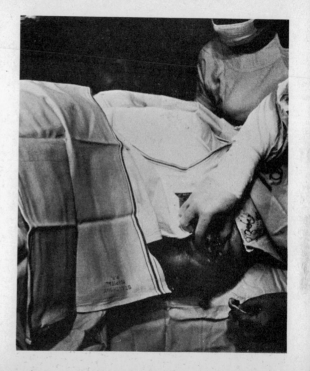

4:45—

Ann pushes with each contraction. When the baby's head "crowns" the doctor tells Ann to stop pushing; she lies back and begins to pant.

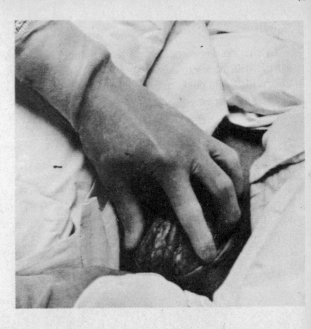

4:50—

The doctor delivers the baby's head, and the most difficult of Ann's task is over.

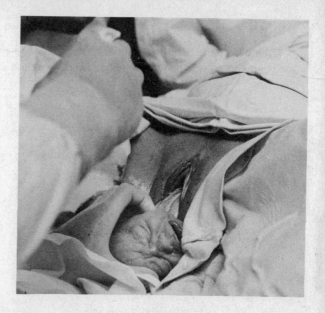

4:55—

Even before the baby is completely born, the doctor begins to suction away the mucus from its mouth and nose.

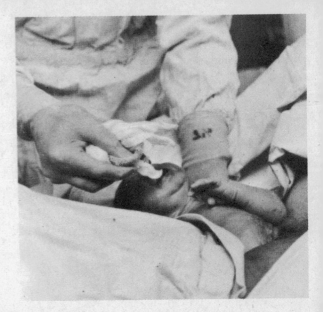

5:00—

The rest of the baby comes effortlessly through the birth canal: a 7½ pound boy.

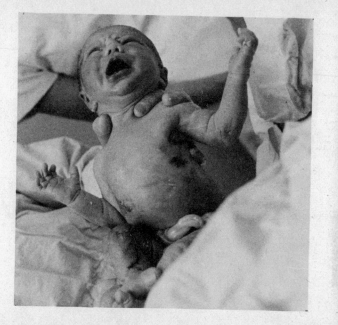

5:10—

Ann eagerly welcomes him: a healthy, beautiful
baby.

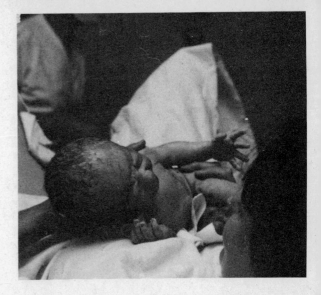

6:00—

Back in the recovery room, Ann and Milt admire their son.

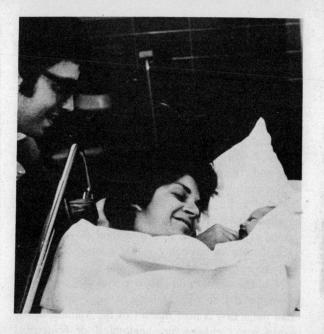

What If Your Labor Isn't "Normal"?

If your labor and delivery progress more or less as described in the preceding chapters, you will have what is called a "normal" labor and delivery. A baby of "normal" size descends in a "normal" position through your "normal" pelvic area in a "normal" amount of time. The training you have received will be of utmost assistance for an endurable and controllable labor and delivery.

But perhaps you are among the minority—your baby is larger than the pelvic outlet or is in an unusual position, or your labor extends over a long period of time for one reason or another—then, let's face it, you are probably in for a long, hard labor and delivery.

Now the question is: "How well will this training serve me if I do run into any of these problems?" You must first realize that all of the training in the world won't change any anatomical or obstetrical

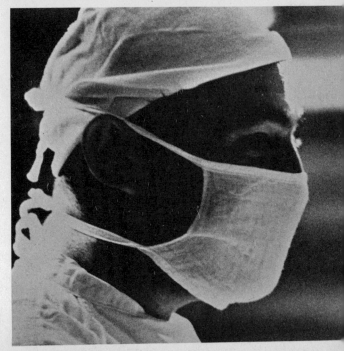

problem. Nor will it help you put your baby in a proper position or eliminate complications in labor. This training will, however, equip you with helpful techniques that make even a difficult labor more comfortable and controllable.

Understanding the mechanics of labor and delivery will help you cooperate knowledgeably with your doctor should a problem arise. If your labor extends over a long period of time, your ability to relax will help you conserve energy that you will need.

Posterior Presentation

One of the most common causes of backaches during labor is the position of the baby. In a "normal" presentation, the soft part of the baby's face is against your tailbone and the hard back of his head against the pubic bone. The soft part gives under the pressure of your spine. If, however, the baby's head is turned "sunny side up," the back of his head is pressing against your tailbone, resulting in discomfort in your back. This low backache is sometimes caused by a breech (buttocks first) presentation. There are three methods to use that may alleviate this pressure on the back: position, temperature, and massage.

Position. The primary rule for back labor is to get the weight and pressure of the uterus off your spine and pelvic area. Usually the best position is to lie on your side, with pillows under your head, uterus, and upper leg. This shifts the weight of the uterus off your back onto the bed. Sometimes a nurse will have you get into the "knee-chest position": put your chest on the bed and get up on your knees.

Temperature. Try both heat and cold. Lie on a heating pad or put a hot washcloth on your lower back. Try an ice-cold pack or washcloth on your back.

Massage. A deep, powerful massage, starting down low on the tailbone and drawn up to the lower back, is most helpful. The stronger the pressure, the more it relieves the discomfort.

Forceps Delivery

If the baby is having a hard time coming down during delivery, your doctor will anesthetize the pelvic area, then insert a hinged instrument called forceps through the vagina, place it carefully around the baby's head, and help him out. Because of the anesthesia, you do not feel the forceps.

Cesarean Birth

Every woman wants to have a normal, uncomplicated pregnancy and to give birth when she is awake and active; however, the chances are now one in ten that she may have her baby delivered by cesarean section. A cesarean delivery may be expected or unexpected. For the unprepared mother a cesarean can be a frightening, disappointing, and depressing experience. However, with preparation, cesarean birth can be a shared, family-centered experience for both the mother and father.

The most common reason for a cesarean is a cephalopelvic disproportion, which means that the baby's head is too large to pass through the pelvis. Another reason for cesarean is malpresentation, that is, a part other than your baby's head is at the cervix. If a baby is premature, or experiences any distress during labor that necessitates immediate delivery, you will probably have a cesarean. If you experience any distress or if contractions are not leading to the baby's birth, your medical caregiver would consider a cesarean birth.

There are two types of cesarean deliveries: the classical section and the low-segment transverse cesarean. A classical section may be performed if you require an emergency cesarean or if the placenta is situated in the lower part of your uterus. The incision is made five inches from the pubis to below the navel through your skin and abdominal muscles. The loose covering membrane is cut to expose the uterus, and a four inch vertical incision is made in the uterus to open it. The membranes lining the uterus are then ruptured and the doctor grasps either your baby's head or feet. After the baby is lifted out, the cord is cut and your baby is given to a medical assistant. The placenta and membranes separate and are delivered through the incision. Your uterus, membranes, and abdominal skin are then closed.

The low segment transverse cesarean is similar but the incision is made horizontally just above your pubic hairline. This procedure is preferable because the incision is made in the section of the uterus that does not contract during labor. Although the total surgery lasts one to one and a half hours, your baby is delivered within the first five to fifteen minutes. The remainder of the time is required to repair the incisions in the uterus and abdominal wall.

Throughout the cesarean section, both you and your coach will be able to use Lamaze techniques. If you go into labor you will want to use the relaxation and breathing techniques to help you cope with contractions. If you do not go into labor you can use these techniques to help you relax before the cesarean. During the cesarean, if you can choose to be awake, you will use your knowledge and information and will know what is happening, for cesarean also means birth—and more importantly, the birth of your baby. After a cesarean you will need to use your breathing and relaxation techniques to help you cope with any pain you may experience. Your coach will use all of the comforting techniques that were learned to help give you relief.

Induction of Labor

Induction of labor means starting the contractions of labor, or increasing the effectiveness of the contractions of labor, through chemical or hormonal medication. Although induction of labor is not necessary in a normal birth, there are times that your medical caregiver may consider induction. Your labor may be induced if your due date has passed and there are indications the baby is post-mature. If contractions during labor are not effective in opening the cervix, you may be given medication to augment, or increase, the intensity of contractions. Whatever the reasons, if labor is induced or augmented, you should be aware that the contractions accompanying induced labor are usually quite strong and more difficult to control.

These are the most common obstetrical complications. If you have any questions, discuss them with your doctor.

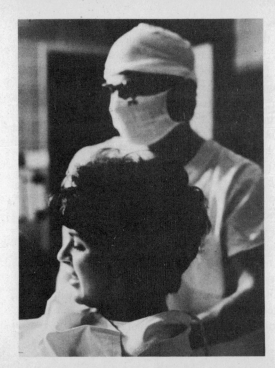

Other Possible Problems That Might Occur During Labor and After Delivery

Hyperventilation

When a woman is breathing too fast, the oxygen and carbon dioxide in her system may get out of balance. If you begin to feel any tingling in your hands, your feet, or the tip of your nose or if you feel any dizziness, you are hyperventilating. Immediately hold your breath (which will permit Nature to restore the balance), or breathe into a small paper bag (you will be re-breathing your own carbon dioxide).

Nausea and Vomiting

Do not eat when you know you are in labor because digestion slows when labor begins. If you do feel nauseous, suck on ice chips, or put a cool washcloth on your throat.

Shivering and Chills

Shivering is a normal bodily response that provides extra warmth. Take in a deep breath between contractions and hold it for five seconds; release as slowly as possible. Repeat several times.

Leg Trembling

Hold your breath between contractions. Release slowly. Have coach hold legs firmly.

Perspiring

Remove extra covers. Place a cool washcloth on forehead.

Sleepiness

Use a cold washcloth on face. Coach, let woman sleep between contractions and wake her up just before the contraction begins so that breathing pattern may be started.

Cramps

Cramps in legs and thighs may be relieved by long, firm stroking of cramp. Do not massage in circles, for that will only increase the cramping. The coach can grasp the woman's foot in his hands, extending the heel toward him and pushing the toes toward the woman's knee while stroking the cramped area.

Hot and Cold Flashes

Put on and take off warm socks and blankets as needed.

Dry Mouth

Ice chips help to moisten mouth; or try a washcloth dipped in cold water and put between lips. Brush teeth.

Backache

Get the woman off her back into a side-lying or knee-chest position. Place hot or cold towels on her back. Massage and counter pressure can also give relief.

Inability to Relax

Coach, take over. Remind woman of the importance of relaxation. Rub back, shoulders, and face. Direct her to change breathing pattern. Emphasize relaxing between contractions. Breathe with her.

Afterbirth Pains

After delivery the nurse must massage your uterus to hasten its return to its normal state; this may be uncomfortable. Your uterus will continue to contract for some time. These contractions are not usually painful with first births. However, with succeeding births the muscle tone of the uterus is less firm and many women feel these contractions very strongly. It sometimes helps to use the light breathing during these contractions.

Stitches

The stitches from the episiotomy are often uncomfortable for the first few days after your delivery. The nurse will usually help you with baths and heat. Your doctor may administer drugs to alleviate discomfort.

Postnatal Blues

Whether it is chemical, emotional, or physical, it happens to the best of us. You are happy with your baby and your husband and everything is wonderful—but you cry at the least provocation and find yourself with the "blues" for no reason at all. It may help to know that this will soon pass.

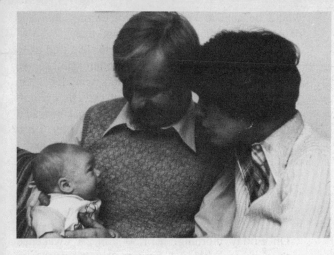

Chapter Eight: Birth Reports

A First Baby

When I became pregnant, I called a few of my friends to see if they could recommend an obstetrician. One of my friends happened to be married to an interning physician, and another friend worked as a medical technologist. Both of them recommended the same doctor, so I called and made an appointment with him.

The day of my appointment arrived. After a thorough examination the doctor and I visited. One of the questions he asked me was if I had ever heard of the Lamaze method of childbirth. I hadn't, and told him so. He explained the method to me briefly. My interest was aroused. My husband and I discussed the method, and decided to enroll in the classes that would teach us the Lamaze technique.

191

We started attending the classes when I was seven months pregnant. The classes were very informative, not only about the Lamaze method, but about birth in general and in detail. I never knew much about birth, but now I was learning what one should expect at the birth of a baby. After a few classes we were taught the basis of the method—relaxing and the breathing exercises. During the next month I practiced relaxing and doing the breathing exercises. My husband Tom was always with me to do the coaching.

During the classes, women who had given birth to children with the Lamaze method came and told about their own experiences with birth. Although no one said it was an extremely easy task, everyone said that the method made birth such a joyful experience. All these women were able to keep themselves in control during labor and delivery. Even though I heard these first-hand reports I was beginning to wonder if all these reports were really true and if I would be able to keep in control during labor and delivery. I had these doubts now and then.

Time was drawing near. The doctor had told us to remember that first babies were often late, so we were resigned to the idea that ours would be. On Wednesday, May 8, I thought that perhaps my amniotic sac was leaking, but I decided that instead I had probably just caught a cold in my bladder. I had an appointment with the doctor on Saturday and I decided I would tell him at that time.

On Thursday I felt fine, just as I had during my whole pregnancy. Tom and I decided to take a leisurely drive in the mountains. We did and enjoyed it.

On Friday morning, at 1:30 a.m., I awakened with a stomach ache. I went to the bathroom and realized that I was having a few contractions—nothing to be excited about, however. They were not strong and were about ten minutes apart. I went back to bed, but my ache persisted, accompanied by diarrhea. At 2:30 my husband awoke and I told him my story. We decided that I was most likely having false labor; besides, I did not want to call the doctor so early in the morning. At 5 a.m. we started to time the contractions and found that they were getting more regular—about five minutes apart. At this time I started the deep chest breathing. By 6:30 the contractions were all about two minutes apart. We called the doctor and he said to leave for the hospital.

At 7 a.m. we arrived at the hospital. Now I was doing the dilatation breathing. I was taken to the prep room and my husband registered me as a patient. I was told that my cervix was two centimetres dilated. Now I was taken to a labor room, where my husband joined me. Time was actually passing very quickly. We were kept very busy. We waited for each contraction. Tom told me when a contraction would be starting, I would do the breathing exercise, and Tom would give me effleurage. Also, Tom would tell me when to expect the apex of the contraction and the end of it. Knowing this seemed to make the contractions pass much more quickly.

The doctor came to examine me about 9:30 a.m. He said that I was doing fine and that the contractions were quite strong.

At 10:30 the doctor came again. My cervix was now four centimetres dilated. The doctor decided that he would give me a paracervical injection to help me relax and perhaps get some rest. Unfortunately, the injection did not take in my case. I was, however, able to stay in control and I continued with my breathing. By now I was not only contending with contractions, but also with hiccups. Tom kept encouraging me. He gave me ice to chew on between contractions and put cool washcloths on my forehead.

Soon I felt the urge to push. I immediately started

my breathing designed for this transitional stage. The doctor came and announced that I was completely dilated. He said that I should start pushing with each contraction.

The delivery of the baby was the easiest part. After four pushes in the delivery room our little girl was born as my husband and I looked on. Kristin Ann, who weighed seven pounds and two ounces, was born at 11:47 a.m. It was a most gratifying and humbling experience.

I am not very good at putting my feelings into words. All I can say is that having a baby is so much easier than I had ever thought it would be. I had our baby with the Lamaze method and I look forward to having another baby the same way. The breathing exercises do work, but they must be practiced beforehand.

I feel that without my husband's help I would not have been able to cope with the situation as well as I did. Husbands certainly play an important role in this method of childbirth.

—Sarah Cornell

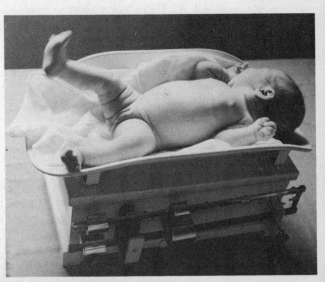

A Second Baby

I am the mother of two children. When my daughter was born, I was given an anesthetic that put me to sleep during most of my labor. What little I remember of that experience was a nightmare. Not only was I frightened but it seemed to me that the anesthesia made me and the baby sick. Every time she was brought to me for feeding, she would throw up. I made up my mind that my next child would be born without my being put to sleep. I couldn't stand the thought of another delivery like that again.

When I suspected that I was expecting another baby, I began asking different friends what type of anesthetic they had been given when their babies were born. Two of my friends were glad to tell me about their experiences. Their babies were born by the Lamaze method of childbirth. The more I heard about the method, the more interested I became. I wanted very much to have my baby this way. I found a doctor who used the method, and signed up for the classes.

My husband was very pleased to learn that he would have an active part in helping me during labor. He had somehow felt cheated over not being allowed to stay with me when our daughter was born. The classes consisted of being told and shown with pictures what happens to a woman during pregnancy and delivery. We were also shown films on actual births—one being a Lamaze birth. One class dealt with the different breathing techniques that are used in the four stages of labor. We were also given typed sheets of paper telling us about the characteristics of these four stages and what the wife's and husband's roles were during each stage. The instructor also showed the husbands how to help their wives relax during labor. She suggested that we should start practicing our exercises at home two or three times a day so that when we did go into labor we would know what to do. I practiced my exercises when my husband was home. My doctor had told me my husband could go with me into the delivery room, so it was important for us to practice those exercises together.

I had what some women refer to as "false labor" off and on the last month of my pregnancy. A week before my baby was born, the contractions bothered me enough so that I went in to see the doctor. He examined me and told me I was effacing but that he felt I would still carry the baby a while longer. The contractions continued all the next week. The night of March sixth was a restless one for me. I couldn't sleep and my contractions were harder than usual, but were not regular. The next morning I had a bloody show. I called my doctor and made an appointment for him to see me that afternoon. My contractions continued but still were not regular. Toward noon I started the deep relaxed chest breathing with the contractions. When I went to the doctor's office at 4:00 p.m. he examined me and told

me I was three centimetres dilated. He told me to return home and when the contractions became regular to call him. Around 6:15 the contractions began to get stronger and regular. I still used the deep chest breathing with these contractions.

By 7:00 p.m. my contractions were about three minutes apart. We called the doctor and started for the hospital. I was pre-registered at the hospital so I was taken directly upstairs to a labor room. I undressed and was examined by the nurse in charge, who in turn told the doctor when he arrived that I was in active labor. I was partially prepped and given an enema. My contractions were quite strong at this time, and I had to concentrate harder on my breathing and relaxing. I switched from the deep relaxed breathing to the shallow breathing. My husband kept reassuring me and helped me with my breathing pattern. I was a little uncomfortable lying on my back, so I switched to a side position which worked better for me. The nurse in charge had seen

Lamaze deliveries before and was a great help. She and my husband kept encouraging me, making sure I stayed relaxed. By that time it was quite hard to do. I began to panic slightly, so I was given an injection to help me relax. I dozed between contractions, and without my husband's help I might have lost control. He timed my contractions and would wake me up before one would start. This way I wasn't caught off guard. Suddenly the contractions became much, much stronger and I was wide awake. I began to breathe a little too fast and became hyperventilated, but with the aid of the nurse we soon had this problem under control.

I was really beginning to doubt my ability to cope with the contractions. My husband kept encouraging me and when the nurse told me I was seven centimetres dilated, I relaxed and tried much harder to concentrate on my breathing and relaxing.

Suddenly I felt a tremendous urge to push. I told the nurse, and you've never seen such a scurry!

Everyone got so excited—everyone but me. I was much too busy breathing and blowing out!

The doctor came in, examined me, gave me a paracervical injection, and instructed the nurse to take me to the delivery room. In the delivery room, I was put on the delivery table and my legs were put in stirrups and draped.

The paracervical anesthetic took away the feeling of pain but I still felt the urge to push. I really had to concentrate so that I wouldn't push too soon. When the doctor told me to push, I breathed in, breathed out, breathed in, breathed out, breathed in, and pushed. The doctor told me to lie back and relax, and then he asked me to push again. I was watching in the mirror over the table and with the second push I saw the baby's head crown. The doctor asked me to lie back again. I did, and began to pant. He performed an episiotomy and then asked me to push again. My husband supported my back while I gave one big push and there was my baby's head, and quite suddenly there was all of my new son. When the doctor cleaned out the baby's nose and mouth, he began to howl vigorously. While the nurses took care of the baby, the doctor asked me to push once more. I did, and the placenta was delivered. I lay back on the table. As far as I was concerned, my work was done. I wanted to hold my baby. I held him for a minute and then the nurse handed him to my husband. Charles smiled and asked me if I wanted to know what time the baby was born. I said yes, and he said "9:15 p.m. I'm glad you didn't lose control, so that I got to be here. I wouldn't have missed this for anything."

What a wonderful fear-free way to have a baby!

—Carolyn Phipps

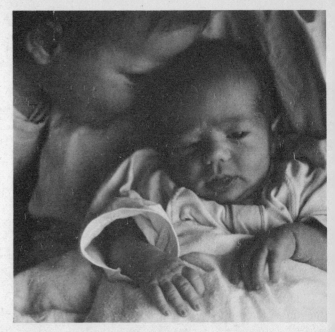

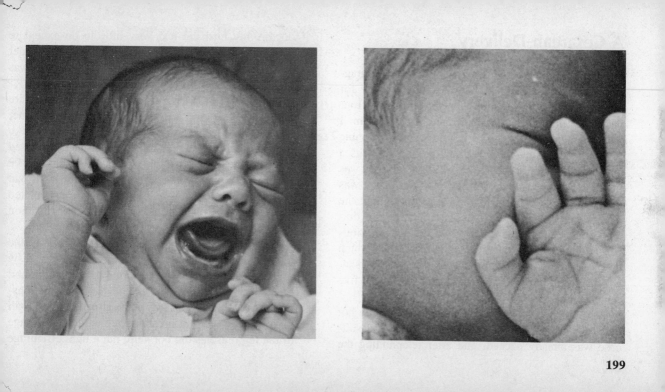

199

A Cesarean Delivery

Two weeks after my due date, my doctor discouragingly announced that the baby wouldn't come for several more weeks. I didn't believe him, and four days later my hunch was confirmed. At 1:00 a.m. I was awakened by cramps in the legs and pubic region, accompanied by a slight feeling of nausea and a brownish-red discharge which I thought was the bloody show (the doctor told me later that it was meconium; it continued to discharge throughout the first stage of labor). I never experienced any dramatic breaking of the waters. During the previous two nights I had felt fairly strong contractions, which disappeared when I got up. These new ones persisted, occurring with reasonable consistency every five minutes and lasting for a minute.

We phoned the doctor, and I took a very long hot bath, which soothed the pains in my legs. My suitcase was already packed, and after telephoning the doctor, my husband had very little to do except to wait for me to emerge from the bath—and to wonder about the drive to the hospital, for although it was mid-May, it was snowing outside.

We arrived at the hospital at 4:30 a.m., and were told that the doctor, expecting us earlier, had come, waited, and then sensibly taken a nap. Because a previous pelvic examination had caused unexpected bleeding the doctor had left word that I was not to be examined, so we had no notion of how far labor had progressed. Expecting a long labor, we speculated the effacement was still in progress and that dilatation had not yet begun.

While still at home, I had been surprised by the intensity of the pain in my legs and discouraged by my inability to control it through relaxation and breathing. After we reached the hospital, my husband and I spent about two hours experimenting with various massage and breathing techniques. Massage of the leg muscles did not help, but a light effleurage was a very effective distraction. Because my abdomen was very sensitive, I did the effleurage myself. A comfortable bed position—with both back and legs slightly raised—was also important. But above all, as time passed, I began to sense the pattern of contractions and could anticipate and breathe with them. Familiarity bred relaxation! I had the impression that the contractions were diminishing in intensity and occurring further apart, neither of which was in fact true. I used deep chest breathing exclusively, and never felt the need for the more shallow and rapid breathing. I was almost totally self-absorbed, and my husband's active participation was quite small, although he was still quite busy with miscellaneous tasks. He gave me a wet washcloth and ice cubes to suck, and timed contractions (with a stop watch, which was extremely handy), letting me know when they were half over. Unfortunately, they were so irregular that he was right only half the time! Nevertheless, the timing was helpful, and had he not been there, my self-confidence—the vital factor—would have suffered badly.

By 7 a.m. we had settled into a comfortable and effective routine and were ready to go on for many hours. Then I was examined, and we were amazed to learn that I was 5 centimetres dilated. We were also surprised, as was the doctor, to discover that the baby was in breech position. I was taken down to the X-ray department to have pelvic photographs taken—contracting, breathing, and relaxing all the way, even on the X-ray table. When I returned to the labor room, the doctor predicted a delivery time of 10 a.m., which I thought was impossible because the contractions felt so mild.

During a subsequent examination, all of our expectations, both pessimistic and optimistic, were shattered. I was found to be fully dilated, having gone from 5 centimetres to this point in an hour. But the baby was poised to come both feet first, with a prolapsed cord in between them. The doctor urgently advised an immediate cesarean section. We were stunned—this was a possibility which we had never considered. But the logic of the case was plain, and we quickly agreed. Both my husband and I had the identical feeling: we each were terribly sorry that the other would not be able to participate in the delivery after all the months of preparation.

Around me pandemonium broke loose, culminating in a hurried trip to the operating room, while my husband was relegated to the waiting room, where he spent three hours before I emerged, barely coherent, from the recovery room. The baby, a girl, was born at 9:58 a.m., and was placed immediately in an incubator. My husband saw her a few minutes later, but because of the effects of anesthetic and operation, I didn't see her until the afternoon of the next day. Two days later, however, I began to nurse her, and two days after that we were able to establish the rooming-in arrangement that we had planned from the start.

My husband and I had begun to investigate various methods of childbirth as soon as I became pregnant. We had read a dozen books, and had participated in classes on the Lamaze technique. We were unusually well prepared, but we were also realistic. Throughout the classes the instructor had stressed, and we agreed completely, that the Lamaze method was not a panacea, but a technique of mental and physical preparation to enable one to cope with both the expected and the unexpected. This attitude was confirmed by my case. The technique took me through to full dilatation with less discomfort than I could have believed, and bolstered my confidence throughout labor. We were able to accept the need for a cesarean section with a maximum of understanding and a minimum of fuss and delay. Our baby, although full term, weighed 4 pounds 6 ounces, and had initial breathing difficulty and very low blood sugar. She might not have survived an attempted normal delivery.

My labor and delivery, to an unusual degree,

represent the best of both the old and the new obstetrical methods. Intensive preparation for childbirth allowed me to remain in full and confident control of the first stage of labor; skilled medical technique carried me—and the baby—the rest of the way when unusual conditions made it necessary to depart from a normal delivery.

—Susan Armitage

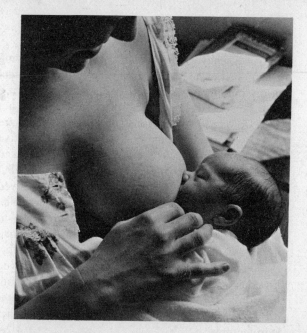

A Father's Report

Until I actually experienced it with my wife, having a baby had always been an abstract process, distant in my mind, vaguely mysterious. Even so, I agreed with her that the routine hospital delivery was not what we wanted. When Nonny discovered the Lamaze class, we gratefully enrolled, hoping for an active experience in which we would be the doers. I looked forward to the birth of our first child, of course, but it was Nonny who felt the growth within, who lived the physical changes. Perhaps because I wasn't to be the one bearing the child, it was easier for me to believe that the technique worked and that all we had to do was practice what we were taught. The information and preparation we received in class proved invaluable when Nonny went into labor; but without my conviction that we could do the Lamaze together, the birth of our girl might have been another story entirely.

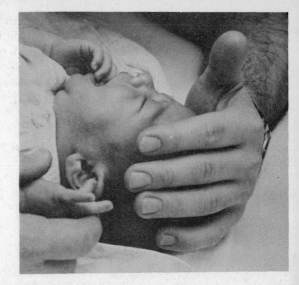

One morning at 2:30, I was sleepily aware that Nonny had been in and out of bed at least a dozen times. Gas, she said. But signs appeared, and a call to the doctor had us preparing for the 40 mile drive to the hospital. Suddenly it was time to practice what we had been conditioned to do: the relaxation, the breathing. Watching her in the rear view mirror, I saw Nonny twist and tighten on the back seat, looks of surprise crossing her face at the intensity of contractions. She was unable to consistently relax or establish a breathing pattern. But the excitement of the high-speed drive to the hospital sustained us both.

Once there, Nonny was wheelchaired out of sight as I signed papers, wrote a check, and parked the car.

Rushing back to the third floor, I couldn't find the Maternity Ward; and when I did, a nurse refused to allow me in the Preparation Room with Nonny.

After ten or fifteen minutes, Nonny emerged and slowly walked to a labor room, and I followed.

She was in bad shape. I had wanted to be with her in the prep room to help her get started with the Lamaze techniques. But by the time I rejoined her, she was an electric knot, twisting and gasping and doubling up like in the movies. "I'm sorry," she said, "but I think I'll have to have a shot . . . and the nurse thinks so, too." The important thing was that she had waited to see me before agreeing to take any drugs. And that required nerve because she was on the verge of losing all control. "We'll try the Lamaze," I said, "you can do it, we're trained and we can do it if we work together." "I don't know, the contractions are so big!" Her contractions didn't stop to allow us time for discussion, but as they became increasingly intense I encouraged her, demanded that she breathe with me, performed the effleurage. As contractions came and went, two things began to happen. Nonny slowly regained control in direct proportion to her degree of relaxation; and I began to *feel* what was happening inside her. We came together, fulfilling separate functions that complemented and truly depended upon one another. A contraction began, we breathed, she relaxed (especially her legs), I rubbed, she bore it, I coaxed her on. After fifteen or twenty minutes we were in control, not really thinking ahead, but dealing with each contraction and preparing for the next. Some were almost overwhelming—it took belief, endurance, and sheer will to get through. At the time, we were unaware that Nonny was in transition and so we continued with dilatation breathing, which was adequate. Between contractions I wiped Nonny's face with a cool washcloth and spooned her ice chips. An hour and a half flashed by as we worked and maintained control. Then the doctor was telling Nonny to push, which gave her tremendous relief and pleasure. Without drugs she had made it to delivery, the easiest and gayest part of the process. Then we anxiously awaited each contraction because our baby was approaching. In the delivery room Nonny's face turned plum-red as she pushed and grinned. When Gabrielle was born at 6:18 a.m., we were all laughing and very happy.

—Jim Ekedahl

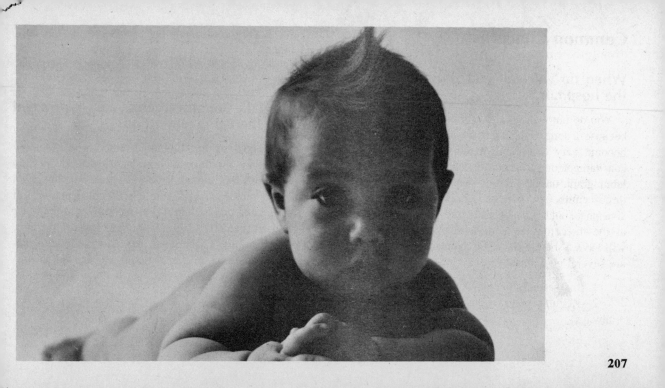

Common Concerns

When do you call your doctor to go to the hospital?

You do not want to arrive at the hospital too early because a long wait in the hospital atmosphere can become very depressing to all those involved and can hamper the progress of your labor. Consult the labor graph on page 81. If you come before two or three centimetres, you are still probably in the passive phase and have hours before you. If you come at the three to four centimetre phase, you usually will have a shorter and more manageable labor. Here are several guidelines:

1. Increasingly intense contractions.
2. Regular contractions (sometimes, but not always).
3. Ruptured membranes (always call your doctor).
4. Contractions three to five minutes apart.

If I take an anesthetic, can I proceed with the Lamaze method?

The goal of the Lamaze method is a "healthy baby," not childbirth without anesthetics. Every doctor knows that the adult dosage of anesthetics given to the mother passes through the placenta in full dosage and can be harmful to the baby. On the other hand, at times (i.e., long labor, prolonged transition, complications, C-sections, lazy uterus, or fetal distress) analgesics and anesthetics are needed to produce a healthy baby.

What can the coach do if the woman loses control?

Do not criticize her. It is not unusual to lose control during the emotional and physical stresses that accompany transition. You must be kind, but very firm, as you get her back into control:

1. Firmly tell her to open her eyes and look at you. Eye contact is very important.
2. Firmly stroke her legs, arms, etc. Concentrate on her breathing.
3. Tell her to breathe in and out with you (she may have forgotten how to breathe) with slow, deep, easy breaths.
4. Have her breathe in and out with you until you feel her gradually begin to relax.
5. As she takes on the breathing pattern herself, you can begin to verbally remind her to relax.
6. Talk to her, give her instructions, give her directions, give her support, give her love.
7. Remind her that the transition is a signal that delivery is not far away and that the more she tenses, the more she will prolong her labor.

What happens if the coach panics during childbirth?

Every coach asks himself, "What if I cannot carry through with this overwhelming responsibility?" Do not worry. The natural process of labor builds slowly, and your ability to cope builds with it. Many men are overwhelmed at the impact of the transitional stage. Remind yourself that the more you can help her relax and remain in control, the shorter the labor will be for both of you. Once you are through transition, the intensity of the contractions seems to diminish, and control and joy once more prevail.

What if the woman is crabby and will not relax?

It is not unusual for a woman to become irritable as labor progresses. If you have practiced during pregnancy, she should be conditioned to relax to your voice and touch. Remind her that the more she can relax, the shorter her labor will be. However, if you find that you are adding to her irritability after trying all the techniques, try to be flexible and understanding. Also, remember that some women have an "irritable uterus" and are disturbed by anyone touching them.

Under what conditions would my coach have to leave the delivery room?

All prepared coaches know that the goal of their preparation is a "healthy baby." Remember that the reasons a coach may be asked to leave will ultimately be for the mother's or baby's health.

1. Complications of mother during delivery: hemorrhaging, C-sections, pelvis too small (pelvic disproportion), or placental problems.
2. Complications for the baby (fetal distress): prolapsed cord, abnormal fetal position, use of forceps, or breech presentation.

How about intercourse during pregnancy? Is it harmful?

Because both the woman and man before the birth of their baby are vulnerable physically and emotionally, sex and lovemaking are essential for the strength of the relationship. If it has been a normal pregnancy, sexual intercourse can be continued to the end. However, the normal position of the man on top can be uncomfortable and unromantic for both the man and woman. This may be a good time to experiment with alternative positions. If any problem or complications arise, be sure to consult your doctor.

What effects do smoking, alcohol, or drugs have on babies?

It is known that all drugs do pass through the placental barrier. It seems to be a matter of quantity rather than of substance. Mothers who smoke heavily do produce smaller babies. Alcoholic mothers can produce alcoholic babies, and drug-addicted mothers can produce addicted babies. Do not take any medications—even the usual household remedies—unless your doctor prescribes them.

Are there any danger signs to be aware of during pregnancy?

Yes; do not hesitate to call your doctor if you develop any of the following symptoms:

1. Bleeding from the vagina—no matter how slight.
2. Swelling of your face, fingers, or ankles.
3. Severe, continuous headaches.
4. Dimness or blurring of vision.
5. Pain in your abdomen.
6. Persistent vomiting.
7. Chills and fevers.
8. Escape of fluid from the vagina.
9. Baby stops moving.

Do coaches have to be in the delivery room?

The woman will work the hardest during labor—this is when she needs you. She needs your directions, your support, and your love. Delivery is the "icing on the cake." The hardest part of the labor is over, and the pushing is usually a joyous relief. If you do not wish to be there, do not feel pressured. However, wait until the actual moment to make the decision. You may be pleasantly relieved to see that at delivery time, pressures decrease and joy and fulfillment increase.

What happens if I must go to the hospital without my coach?

This is a normal concern and happens to a very small percentage of patients. However, anyone benefits by having knowledge, training, and techniques to carry them through labor and delivery. If possible, find a friend, mother, or sister to give you support.

Is practice really necessary, and if so, how often?

Lamaze means practice. An Olympic racer would not perform without practice. Labor and delivery are the hardest tasks you will perform—do not go into them without practice or you will be sorely disappointed with the results. Education is not enough.

Practice your relaxation and breathing exercise at least twice daily: once in the morning by yourself and once in the evening with your coach.

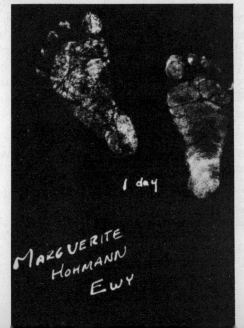

1 day

MARGUERITE
HOHMANN
EWY

Further Reading

General

The Art of Loving. Erich Fromm. Harper and Row, 1967.

Our Bodies, Ourselves. Boston Women's Health Book Collective. Simon & Schuster, 1976.

Pregnancy

Essential Exercises for the Childbearing Year. Elizabeth Noble. Houghton Mifflin, 1976.

The First Nine Months of Life. Geraldine L. Flanagan. Simon & Schuster, 1962.

Is My Baby All Right? Virginia Apgar and Joan Beck. Trident, 1973.

Life Before Birth. Ashley Montague. New American Library, 1964.

Making Love During Pregnancy. Elisabeth Bing and Libby Colman. Bantam, 1977.

Pregnancy: The Psychological Experience. Libby Colman and Arthur Colman. Herder and Herder, 1972.

Childbirth

Awake and Awake. Irwin Chabon. Delacorte, 1969.

The Caesarean Birth Experience. Bonnie Donovan. Beacon Press, 1977.

The Experience of Childbirth. Sheila Kitzinger. Pelican, 1972.

Have It Your Way. Vicki Walton. Bantam, 1978.

Thank You, Dr. Lamaze. Marjorie Karmel. Doubleday, 1965.

Why Natural Childbirth? Deborah Tanzer and Jean Block. Schocken, 1976.

Childbirth without Pain. Dr. Pierre Vellay. E.P. Dutton & Co., 1960.

Painless Childbirth through Psychoprophylaxis. Dr. Isadore Bonstein. William Heinemann Medical Books, Ltd., 1958.

Six Practical Lessons for an Easier Childbirth. Elisabeth Bing. R.P.T. Grosset & Dunlap, 1967.

Training Manual. Elisabeth Bing and Marjorie Karmel. A.S.P.O., 1967.

The New Childbirth. Erna Wright. Hart Publishing Co., 1966.

Nutrition and Breastfeeding

The Complete Book of Breastfeeding. Marvin Eiger and Sally Olds. Bantam, 1973.

Natural Baby Food Cookbook. Margaret Kenda and Phyllis Williams. Nash, 1972.

Nourishing Your Unborn Child. Phyllis Williams. Nash, 1974.

Nursing Your Baby. Karen Pryor. Pocket Books, 1973.

Preparation for Breastfeeding. Donna Ewy and Rodger Ewy. Doubleday, 1975.

The Tender Gift: Breastfeeding. Dana Raphael. Schocken, 1976.

What Every Pregnant Woman Should Know. Faith Brewer and Tom Brewer. Random House, 1977.

Childcare and Parenting

Child Care. Sutherland Learning Associates, Inc. 1973.

The First Twelve Months of Life. Frank Caplan. Grosset & Dunlap, 1973.

The Growth and Development of Mothers. Angela McBride. Harper and Row, 1973.

How to Parent. Fitzhugh Dodson. Signet, 1970.

Infants and Mothers—Differences in Development. T. Berry Brazelton. Dell, 1972.

The Magic Years. Selma Fraiberg. Scribner's, 1959.

Maternal—Infant Bonding. Marshall Klaus and John Kennell. C.V. Mosby Co., 1976.

Parent Effectiveness Training. Thomas Gordon. McKay, 1970.

Preparing for Parenthood. Lee Salk. Bantam, 1975.

What Now? A Handbook for New Parents. Mary Lou Rozdilsky and Barbara Banet. Scribner's, 1975.

What To Do When There's Nothing To Do. Elizabeth Gregg. Dell, 1970.

If these books are not available at your local bookstore, they may be ordered from:

Birth and Life Bookstore, Inc.
P.O. Box 70625
Seattle, WA 98107

International Childbirth Education Association, Inc. (ICEA)
P.O. Box 20048
Minneapolis, MN 55420

Resources

Listing of Parents' Organizations

American National Red Cross
    17th & D Streets
    Washington, DC 20006
American Society for Psychoprophylaxis in Obstetrics (ASPO)
    1411 K Street, N.W.
    Washington, DC 20005
Caesarean/Support, Education and Concern (C/SEC, INC.)
    15 Maynard Road
    Dedham, MA 02026
International Childbirth Education Association (ICEA)
    P.O. Box 20852
    Milwaukee, WI 53220

La Leche League
    9616 Minneapolis Avenue
    Franklin Park, IL 60131
Maternity Center Association
    48 East 92nd Street
    New York, NY 100028
National Association of Parents and Professionals for Safe Alternatives in Childbirth (NAPSAC)
    P.O. Box 267
    Marble Hill, MO 63764
National Sudden Infant Death Syndrome Foundation
    310 S. Michigan Avenue
    Chicago, IL 60640
U.S. Consumer Product Safety Commission
    Washington, DC 20207
    800-492-2937

Audiovisual Programs

Educational Graphic Aids, Inc.
  1315 Norwood Avenue
  Boulder, CO 80302
  (303) 449-8049

Index

NOTES

NOTES